Early Praise for *Beating Asthma*

"Beating asthma is a great guide for the asthma patient seeking answers and wanting more control. It's fact-based and reflects the experience of a master physician—if you follow the 'seven P's,' you will go a long way toward taking back control of your life."

—*Dr. Bob Lanier, Fellow, American College of Allergy, Asthma & Immunology; Fellow, American Academy of Allergy, Asthma & Immunology*

"Dr. Apaliski's passion for patient care and education jump off every page of his book. Clearly, all asthma patients will benefit greatly from reading his book cover to cover and following his advice. This is also an excellent resource for anyone who provides care to asthma patients and I know it will hold a prominent place on my bookshelf!"

—*Dr. Bill Berger, Past President, American College of Allergy, Asthma, & Immunology; Author, Asthma for Dummies*

"Dr. Apaliski's seven principles clearly outline the steps for 'fighting' asthma and winning the battle. This book clearly and concisely covers all the aspects of asthma care that I wish I could teach my patients at each visit but don't have the time to do. It's a must-read if you are serious about 'beating' asthma."

—*Dr. Michael Blaiss, Past President, American College of Allergy, Asthma, & Immunology*

"Knowing what my triggers are, and how I can minimize my exposure when appropriate, affords me a more active, healthy lifestyle with asthma. This book is a great resource for my toolbox as I learn to gain control of my asthma. Who am I kidding? This book is a great resource for anyone with asthma!"

—*Ronald (Andy) Carroll, Asthma Patient*

"Truly outstanding...beneficial to patients and their families and a wonderful educational tool."

— *Suzi Grant, Asthma Patient*

"Dr. Apaliski's patient-centered approach to the practice of medicine continually shines through this extremely helpful guide. His long-term experience caring for asthma patients has allowed him to simplify a complex disease, in a text that can be helpful either via a one time 'sit-down read' or as a reference used to answer specific questions."

— *Dr. Phil Lieberman, Past President, American Academy of Allergy, Asthma & Immunology*

Beating Asthma

Beating Asthma

Seven Simple Principles

Stephen Apaliski, MD

Ad majorem Dei gloriam.

Contents

Foreword... xi

Introduction 1

1 Asthma in America.. 7

2 Your Secret Formula for Fighting Asthma:
   Meet the Seven "P" Principles 21

3 Understanding the Problem 39

4 Prevention by Avoidance: Mites, Pollens, and Molds........... 49

5 Prevention by Avoidance: Non-Allergic Triggers 61

6 Pulmonary Function Tests... 71

7 Pharmaceuticals 85

8 The Asthma Action Plan 109

9 The Patient–Physician Relationship................................. 119

10 Positive Mindset... 133

   Conclusion: How the Seven Principles Work 143

   Appendices... 149

   Appendix A: Additional Resources 151

Appendix B: Asthma Action Plans:
Further Comments and Resources 153

Appendix C: Tools to Evaluate
Your Asthma Control.. 157

Appendix D: When to See an Allergist................................ 159

Appendix E: How to Use Asthma Inhalers 163

Notes 165

Acknowledgements 169

About the Author.. 175

Foreword

Everyone knows someone with asthma. Most times it is a bothersome but not dangerous disease. But about fifteen people will die from asthma today and every day this year. Those unfortunate individuals with asthma include successful and well-educated people as well as the urban poor and everyone in between. There is no discrimination for race, creed, religion, education level, geographic location, or other concomitant health issues. These facts are part of the reasons why asthma is included as one of the five major targets for control by so many health agencies from every perspective, ranging from the economic costs to the staggering hospitalization rate and morbidity of this common disease. Thus, asthma warrants our attention and if you or a family member has asthma, this book offers you important and relatively simple lessons on how to survive and thrive, despite having asthma.

The understanding of asthma has undergone a sea change over the past forty years, and as a result the medications available and the medical approaches to asthma have become far more effective than ever before. Then why do asthmatic individuals still get admitted to the hospital and die at such an alarming rate? The data say that most asthma patients are not cared for by specialists, do not get educated about their disease, and are not receiving the proper medications for their degree of severity. As Dr. Apaliski so clearly points out, most patients have an extremely poor perception of the degree of severity of their disease and most are being treated by non-specialists with inappropriate medications. In fact, one third of all the individuals with asthma who will die today have relatively mild asthma. These seemingly healthy patients get sick with either an infection or allergy attack and don't know what to do or how to assess the severity of their attack. They do not have an action plan, do not have a well-trained asthma specialist to call, and their disease worsens before they get care. For those who will die today, that care is either too little or too late.

Anyone who reads Dr. Apaliski's fine book will understand how to assess their disease and will receive the proper foundation of what to do should they get sick. I especially like his comments that all of us who specialize in asthma care welcome sick calls because we realize that early intervention is not only essential but that it can be lifesaving. Dr. Apaliski's simple, straightforward lessons are easily understood and applied, and they can save you or your loved one's lives. I concluded once I had read this book that I would purchase a number of copies for my office staff to read in order to help us apply the principles and lessons contained in *Beating Asthma*.

Thus, it is a pleasure to welcome this book to our medical library, and I recommend it to every asthmatic individual and their family. Those of you reading this foreword are taking an important first step to ensuring your asthma health. Please read on.

Michael A. Kaliner, MD
Medical Director, Institute for Asthma & Allergy
Wheaton and Chevy Chase, MD
Former President, Academy of Allergy, Asthma & Immunology
and the World Allergy Organization

Introduction

"Now this is not the end. It is not even the beginning of the end.
But it is, perhaps, the end of the beginning."

—Winston Churchill

Asthma cannot be cured, but it can be *beaten*. What do I mean by this?

Achieving the best control of asthma possible *for you* is *beating asthma*. I believe you can achieve this goal! That is why I have written this book.

Millions of people struggle with asthma that is not well controlled. So you are not alone, even though you may feel this way at times. Although asthma can kill, and does, most of the suffering it produces is by disrupting the normal rhythm and flow of daily life. Sleep disturbance, Emergency Room (ER) visits, missed school and work, and interference with physical activity are some of the ways that uncontrolled asthma may affect your life. As a result, it may rob you of the quality of life you desire and deserve.

This book provides you with a framework for understanding asthma at a deeper level.

How?

By helping you understand and apply seven simple, powerful, and practical principles that are used by allergy physicians—that is, asthma specialists—and their patients, to successfully improve their quality of life.

The best asthma outcomes are seen in patients who are treated by asthma specialists. Yet, with over 20 million asthma sufferers in the United States and only 4,000 allergists, it is impossible for all asthmatics to be under the care of an asthma specialist. I believe the answer lies in empowering you.

Over the past two decades, there have been great efforts made at educating physicians about the best ways to treat asthma, but evidence suggests that this information and effort is not having a significant impact. I believe that by helping *you* understand the important points of asthma treatment, we can make a difference together. By knowing what is important regarding the treatment of your asthma and what to expect as the standard of care, you will accept nothing less. This will transform you into your own best advocate.

To illustrate, take a little side trip with me for a moment. Think about automobile maintenance. If a healthy, well-functioning car is the desired outcome, how is it that this goal will be best reached? Will it be when the automotive technician has the knowledge of what needs to be done to maintain your vehicle's health but doesn't take the time to teach it to you? Or, is it a collaborative effort, where you are educated about the steps that need to be taken to keep your car healthy and then you make certain that these steps are executed in a timely fashion using a competent mechanic?

Most of us would agree that the best results are obtained in the second scenario. You don't have to know how to change the oil, rotate the tires, do an alignment, or adjust the timing yourself. But, if you know *what* needs to be done and *when*, you will be better able to serve as a good partner with your mechanic in maintaining your vehicle in the best of health.

So it is with asthma. I have seen it thousands of times. Patients who do the best in controlling and beating asthma are those who understand and apply these seven simple principles.

They are simple, but their application is not always easy. They involve work. In the end, though, it is worth the effort. Through these principles, you will know what to expect and be able to request what you need from your physician to properly treat your asthma. You will also develop the confidence to seek a new physician, if necessary, to work with you on this journey.

I write this book as an asthma expert. I have been a practicing physician for over thirty years. I trained as a pediatrician at Children's Hospital of Pittsburgh and later as an allergist at Wilford Hall United States Air Force Medical Center in San Antonio, Texas. I have been blessed with many excellent teachers. I can honestly say that my best teachers have been the many patients who have trusted me as a partner in their healthcare over the years. At their side, I have seen miraculous wins and devastating losses. I have laughed and cried and dreamed with them. To paraphrase the words of Jack Nicholson's character in the movie *As Good As It Gets*, "You make me want to be a better man (physician)!" For this opportunity to grow, learn, help, and support, I remain eternally grateful to my patients.

So, off we go! First, we will review the state of asthma in America. Next, we will look at an overview of the seven principles, followed by individual chapters devoted to each: Problem, Prevention, Pulmonary Function Tests, Pharmaceuticals, Plan, Patient–Physician Relationship, and Positive Mindset.

Each chapter is intended to help you learn a little bit more about how to control your asthma, once and for all.

Controlled asthma is beaten asthma. My hope and prayer for each of you is that you are able to reach this welcome state and improve the quality of your life so that you can live your days to the fullest.

This is, as Winston Churchill put it, the end of the beginning. Beating asthma is a journey, and I want to personally invite you to *not* go it alone. Instead, I invite you to become part of the Beating Asthma community at www.beatingasthma. com. This book is a starting point. You can turn to the Beating Asthma website for additional conversation, information, updates, and more to help you on your way to beating asthma. Together, we can help you return to leading your life the way that you want to live it—active, hopeful, productive, happy, and free of fear!

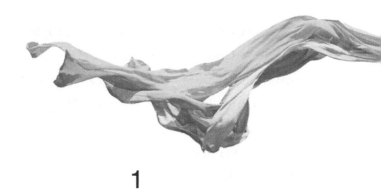

1

Asthma in America

I had come to know Sarah* over the years as a typical pre-teenager. She was energetic, bright, unabashedly honest, and full of life. She never seemed to let her asthma get her down. In short, she was a great kid.

Beaten by asthma, Sarah died on Father's Day.

Never having lost a child, I could only imagine the deep pain her parents felt. Devastated. Crushed. Defeated. I saw the deep sadness in her father's eyes and felt the pain in his voice. As her physician, I found that Sarah's death left a scar within me—a never-healing mark that is still there to this day.

---

* In order to protect identities and confidentiality, all patient names used in this book have been changed.

Sarah became one of almost 4,000 people to die from asthma in the United States that year. Although this number is down from a high of over 5,000 yearly deaths twenty years ago, I believe that it is still unacceptable. We need to do better as a healthcare community—for promising young people like Sarah and for her heartbroken mom and dad.

As bad as these numbers are, they only tell a small part of the story of suffering from asthma. Why? There are actually over 22 million people with asthma in the United States today, and many of them are having a tough time.

HOW BAD CAN ASTHMA GET?

You may be living with asthma that is causing problems and just accepting it as the way it is. Perhaps you are missing school or work, athletic events, or having nights of interrupted sleep from coughing and wheezing. In cases like the last, other family members are oftentimes awakened as well (especially when a child is involved)—so the quality and amount of everyone's sleep and rest are affected!

Not only is the quality of your life lowered by these asthma consequences, but you are also exposed to the risk of death. That's frightening, isn't it? But I don't want you to have to be frightened—that is one of the reasons I am writing this book. Fortunately, death due to asthma is uncommon, though asthma patients and their families face a reduced quality of life way too often.

In 2009, a large survey called Asthma Insight and Management (AIM) was conducted in the United States. It provided an excellent understanding of the impact of this disease in a sample of 2,500 patients with asthma.*

To me, the most striking piece of information gathered in this survey was this: when asked to describe their asthma, 71% of patients reported it to be well or completely controlled. Yet, when asked about specific problems (such as frequency of symptoms, interference with normal activity, and use of bronchodilators and oral steroids), the answers showed that only 29% of them were well controlled. Seventy-one percent, in fact, could be described as *poorly controlled*!

Why would so many patients with asthma believe that their asthma is under control when it is not? The answer to this question is not 100% clear; yet we must consider that this discrepancy occurs as a result of low expectations for what asthma control really looks like. These patients may well be settling for less wellness than they deserve.

Looking at medication use, many people (41%) who had been prescribed long-term asthma medications reported in the AIM study that they had stopped this medication for a week or longer in the past year; 23% reported that they had

---

* The AIM study (www.takingaimatasthma.com) looked at more than 2,000 adults and 300 children with asthma. Interviews were also performed with approximately 1,000 adults without current asthma, and more than 300 physicians. Advisors to this survey included Drs. Michael Blaiss, Eli Meltzer, Kevin Murphy, Robert Nathan, and Stuart Stoloff.

stopped for a month or longer! This approach to medication can cause problems. Stopping these meds places you at greater risk for a more severe asthma attack in the following months. While research is being done on the intermittent use of medications to treat asthma, this approach is not currently widely recommended.

The AIM survey also reported that many asthma patients experience moderate to extremely bothersome symptoms. Even more alarming, one out of three asthma patients also reported the need for acute care for their illness in the past year, including visits to the Emergency Room and hospitalization. Think middle-of-the-night asthma attack with no ability to breathe, ending in a scary mad dash to the ER. That's not the picture of asthma you should settle for.

What did the AIM study reveal about the *treatment* of asthma? Although asthma is its own disease with a unique host of causes, symptoms, and outcomes, primary care physicians—rather than specialists—provide most of the care for asthma! I have a deep regard for primary care doctors, who bear the lion's share of healthcare in America and who help patients get back on the road to wellness day after day. Yet, certain health conditions require specialized care. Unless we provide additional training in this regard to primary care physicians, asthma care by specialists (allergists and pulmonologists) will likely continue to yield the best outcomes.

AIM found that 48% of asthma patients *never* see an asthma specialist—or see one only if problems occur (15%).

Thankfully, there have been some small positive changes in certain areas of asthma care and treatment over the years, shown when one compares the AIM findings with a previous survey completed eleven years earlier—for example, small decreases in the need for acute care, and the days of school or work missed because of asthma. Yet, these changes have been relatively minor.[1] Overall, there hasn't been an improvement in asthma *outcomes*, especially the degree to which asthma sufferers are using emergency care to address their asthma symptoms.

Taking all this in, one might be tempted to feel hopeless; but focusing on the problems we have will only lead us in the wrong direction. As a doctor, I see hope everywhere I look. I have seen many children and adults who previously had multiple hospitalizations for asthma and many visits to the Emergency Room gain control over their disease and never need emergency care or hospital stays for asthma attacks again. I have seen stressed parents who did not know how to handle things become educated and confident, breaking the grip that asthma had on their lives. I see hope in the changes that can and do occur in individual lives.

Yes, there is still much work to do, but I believe we can accomplish that work by finding solutions one person at a time. In the end, it is empowerment that leads to action and action that is the key to solving these problems, enabling you to beat asthma.

ASTHMA OUT OF CONTROL VERSUS UNDER CONTROL

Although each person's asthma takes on its own form and character, two distinct groups emerge among the asthmatic population: those who have uncontrolled asthma versus those who have controlled asthma. This book will help you determine which camp you (or your child) are in so you can see what gaps you may or may not be experiencing in your current treatment plan.

Please don't worry if you find that your (or your child's) asthma is uncontrolled. Remember: Knowledge is power. Realizing the uncontrolled state of your asthma is the first step to improving it!

Uncontrolled asthma. Let's look at the face of uncontrolled asthma. When asthma is not controlled, it is, in fact, *in control* of your life. Chaos may be a good way to describe it. Coughing, wheezing, and chest tightness occur often. As noted earlier, sleep is often interrupted by these symptoms, and maybe even several times a night. On top of the nighttime disruption, life's daily routine is interrupted by unplanned visits to the doctor for emergency care. Children are absent from school, adults from work, and full participation in many activities becomes impossible.

In children, lung growth may be affected, and in adults, lungs may become damaged due to asthma. This is all quite disturbing to say the least. In fact, the AIM study found that 36% of patients at some time had an asthma attack so severe that they were worried that their life was in danger. Thirteen percent of those surveyed reported that they had felt this way within the past year.

For those with uncontrolled asthma, a general feeling of helplessness may also rule their lives. In turn, helplessness may lead to hopelessness, a very dark place to be indeed. Again, the AIM study found that, compared to people without asthma, people with asthma are more likely to feel isolated or alone, fearful, depressed or blue, embarrassed, and angry. Can we blame them? It's no surprise that daily and nightly disruptions to a function as essential as breathing would be deeply upsetting.

My experience tells me that people with controlled asthma are less likely to carry this emotional baggage. I see the smiling faces of the children with controlled asthma in my office and their parents, who no longer have worry lines on their foreheads or circles under their eyes. I get to make small talk with my adult patients with controlled asthma, because their care is going so smoothly. So there's hope. When we bring asthma under control, we are likely to relieve not just its physical burden but its psychological burden as well.

Controlled asthma. Now, let's look at life with controlled asthma. If you fall into this camp, you are only reaching for your short-acting bronchodilator inhaler once or twice a week, if at all. You are sleeping through the night without interruptions to your breathing. You are attending work or school, and even participating in exercise or athletic events. Quite simply, when asthma is controlled, *you* are back in control of your life. Gone for the most part are the chaotic and upsetting events that those with uncontrolled disease regularly face. Life is more predictable—calmer—and because of this, a certain serenity may be found.

People with controlled asthma are meeting the goals of asthma therapy as set forth in the National Heart, Lung, and Blood Institute (NHLBI for short) Expert Panel's "Asthma Guidelines." What are these goals? They are divided into those that reduce impairment from current asthma problems and those that reduce the risk of future problems, as shown in the textbox that follows. (In my mind, reducing impairment *does* reduce risk!)

Asthma Can Be Controlled

Scientific evidence clearly shows that most people could control their asthma by following current asthma clinical practice guidelines. With proper care, people who have asthma can stay active, sleep through the night, and avoid having their lives disrupted by asthma attacks.

As a general rule, patients with well-controlled asthma have:

- few, if any, asthma symptoms
- few, if any, awakenings during the night caused by asthma symptoms
- no need to take time off from school or work due to asthma
- few or no limits on full participation in physical activities
- no Emergency Room visits
- no hospital stays
- few or no side effects from asthma medicines.

Figure 1. From the National Heart, Lung, and Blood Institute's "Asthma Guidelines."[2]

Attaining these goals is what you are reaching for! Reaching them means different things to each of you.

The takeaway from this is a sense of how stark a difference exists between controlled and uncontrolled asthma. I want you to see that if you are struggling with uncontrolled asthma, there is something much better waiting for you. You *can* get your asthma under control, and what a life awaits you when you do!

A HANDY GUIDE FOR ASSESSING ASTHMA

What do you use as a patient (or parent) to determine where your asthma (or child's asthma) stands? Are there some tools out there that are easy to commit to memory and use? Thankfully, the answer is yes.

Dr. Mark Millard, a Pulmonary Specialist who practices in the Baylor Healthcare System in Dallas, Texas, developed the "Rules of Two" assessment as a quick, easy-to-use test that allows you to determine where your asthma stands. There are four easy questions to remember, and each question involves the number two, hence, the "Rules of Two." (I have made a minor alteration, substituting the word *bronchodilator* for the term *quick-relief medication*.) The questions are shown in the following text box.

Rules of Two®

- Do you have asthma symptoms or use your bronchodilator medication more than two times per week?
- Do you have asthma symptoms that awaken you more than two times per month?
- Do you refill your bronchodilator medication more than two times per year?
- Does your peak flow level drop more than 20% (2x10%)?

If the answer to each of these questions is no, then most likely your asthma is under control. Keep doing what you are doing! A yes answer to one of these questions means that your asthma is not controlled and you need to take action to fix it.

Used with permission of Baylor Health Care System.

Here you have a simple, but powerful tool to let you know how your asthma is doing. This tool empowers you. (Hint: Go to www.beatingasthma.com to download a free reminder card of the "Rules of Two" to keep with you and share with others.)*

---

* There are other tools to help evaluate the question of asthma control, such as the Asthma Control Test (ACT), in which you answer a number of questions, the answers are scored, and, then, based upon your total score, your asthma is classified as controlled or uncontrolled. I have included an explanation of and a URL for taking the ACT in an appendix at the back of this book.

If you monitor your asthma on a weekly and then monthly basis using the Rules of Two, you are less likely to be blindsided and surprised by asthma suddenly being out of control. You will see problems developing and take action. And the sooner you act, the better off you will be—problems with asthma tilting out of control are easier to take care of soon after they begin, rather than after they have gone downhill for some time without action. We will see the "Rules of Two" again in future chapters, along with some other simple tools (such as the Asthma Control Test), all aimed at helping you monitor and take charge of your disease.

We have covered a lot of information in this chapter. If you are battling asthma, you know that you are not alone. Many people are struggling with this disease. Uncontrolled, asthma ends up controlling your life. Gaining control of asthma puts you back in charge of your life. At the time of this book's printing, we are not yet able to cure asthma, but, in most cases, it can be better managed. Believe me, you can do it, too. I see it happen every day.

As an example, I remember a single mom who had recently moved to Texas. She had a young toddler with asthma and was visiting the Emergency Room with him often because he was waking up several times a week at night and needing frequent breathing treatments. As you can imagine, neither the mom nor her son were getting the rest they needed. In addition, she was stressed by the recent move, her new job, and her son's asthma. Chaos.

This mom brought her son in for evaluation. We worked together over the course of a few months to get his asthma under control. When she returned to see me six months later, I was gratified by the change! Gone were the Emergency Room visits. Gone were the frequent nighttime episodes. Mom also had a calmness and relaxed demeanor that I had not seen when we first met. She gained control over her son's disease, and her life was transformed! She told me I was her hero (blush).

The fact is, she was the heroine. She came for help and took action. I couldn't do it for her; she had to do it for herself and for her son. And do it she did, like a star. Happily, her son's story of improvement is not the exception; it is the rule. When you manage this disease to the best extent possible as she and many others do, you are indeed beating asthma.

Now, onto the next chapter where I will introduce you to seven principles that will help turn you into the asthma-beating dynamo that I know you can be.

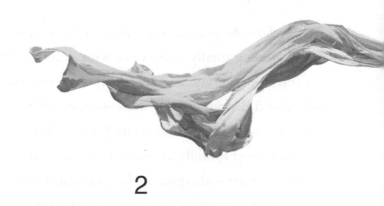

2

Your Secret Formula for Fighting Asthma: Meet the Seven "P" Principles

Is there a way to get back to a normal life when you have asthma?

Is it possible to give the bronchodilator inhaler a little rest? Is it possible to go to bed at night without worry about waking from an attack? Can you (or your child) actually get back to playing sports again? The answer is yes. All these things and more are possible. For those of you with severe asthma, there is also hope for fewer ER visits, fewer hospitalizations, and—if time in the hospital is necessary—shorter stays. This is good news!

But how do you get from here to there? Some of you may be feeling totally exasperated with asthma. Although I can't offer you a magic wand to simply wave over your asthma and make it disappear, I do have some powerful information that can change your and your family's life. Think of it as the allergist's secret formula for successful asthma care.

Don't worry—allergists are not concerned about keeping you from discovering this secret formula. It's not really a secret. I want to help get the word out about the allergist's approach to asthma so that you can start getting the most out of life.

ASTHMA SPECIALISTS VS. GENERALIST PHYSICIANS

Why should anyone care about how allergists treat asthma?

As it turns out, *asthma specialists* tend to have better results when working with asthma patients than do *primary care doctors*. It's not that we asthma specialists are any brighter than our primary care colleagues—it's just that we've had the benefit of specialized training in the realm of asthma.

In a publication from the American College of Allergy, Asthma & Immunology in 2009, editors Michael Foggs, MD, and Bradley Chipps, MD, presented data from dozens of published medical studies and reports that support the existence of superior outcomes for patients who have their asthma managed by an asthma specialist rather than a generalist physician.[1] For example, patients report higher ratings of quality of care, improved physical functioning, and improved quality of life. These data also showed that care by asthma specialists results in a 77% reduction in hospitalizations, a 45% reduction in sick-care office visits, a 77% reduction in time lost from work or school, a 95% reduction in inpatient care costs, and a 77% reduction in Emergency Room costs compared to general care physicians! It certainly appears that your quality of life can't help but improve when you work with an asthma specialist.

The National Heart, Lung, and Blood Institute, which regularly issues and updates NIH's Asthma Guidelines, recognizes the need for specialty care for patients with asthma that is difficult to control. In fact, Foggs and Chipps pointed to a study that revealed that in those primary care physicians who had some dedicated training in allergic diseases such as asthma, 78% referred patients to an allergist in contrast to 46% who were less educated about this!

Am I trying to bash primary care physicians? No, I respect my primary care colleagues very much. I am instead pointing out the likelihood that, if you are a primary care physician who doesn't fully understand or appreciate what a specialist physician does and how they can help patients, you may be less inclined to include them in your "toolbox."

If circumstances or your own preferences mean working with a generalist physician, this book can serve as a roadmap for your work together. As you will discover in Chapter 9 on the patient–physician relationship, I believe it is essential that you work with a doctor who is open to learning from you and who is willing to have you be an active partner in your care.

I have spent the past twenty-four years as an allergist pondering these things. What is it about what I and my colleagues in allergy do that is different? What is there in our approach that matters, and how can we get this information to people who need it? Is there a framework we can provide to people with asthma that is simple but effectively points the way to the basic principles needed to empower them and help them to beat asthma?

Enter the Seven "P" Principles. These principles are not intended to be encyclopedic in scope, but they do illustrate the seven touchstones that I believe are essential in helping you beat this disease. They are intended to help you understand what must be addressed if your asthma is to be controlled as best as it can be. They are, from what I have seen over the years, the common elements employed by specialists in caring for their patients with asthma. They are secret in the sense that although known by some, they have not been shared with all asthma sufferers in this way. I will cover each principle briefly here and devote a chapter to each of them after this.

1. UNDERSTANDING THE PROBLEM

If you have an understanding of the nature of asthma, you can begin to discover how to better manage it.

Asthma is a chronic disease of the lungs that involves tightening of the muscles that surround the airways or breathing tubes in the lungs. Excess mucus is produced in those who have asthma, and the airways themselves become inflamed. Although it is not always clear what causes asthma, we do know that various elements (e.g., allergens, viruses, and irritants) entering the lungs play a role in causing these reactions to occur. When lungs react this way, they can be described as "twitchy" or "reactive."

In a person with asthma, the lungs are prone to functioning in a compromised state, resulting in coughing, wheezing, shortness of breath, and chest tightness. For reasons that we don't yet fully understand, the lungs in a person with asthma tend to be more disadvantaged at nighttime, thus there can be the nighttime problems we have already discussed.

Remember these key words—chronic, mucus, muscle tightening, inflammation, and twitchiness—and you will know the essentials. Let's look at two patients with asthma as examples.

Take Larry, an adult with asthma. From Larry's perspective, his asthma involved problems that seemed to occur every month or so. He seemed to get a cold and then his chest would have tightness, a terrible cough, and wheezing. In response, Larry would treat himself with over-the-counter medicines.

Several times a year, things would get so bad for Larry that he would have to go to the Emergency Room or Urgent Care Center near his home for treatment. He would then take the prescribed medicines for a few days, but as soon as he felt better, he would stop them. In his mind, Larry had asthma when he was feeling bad, and when he felt better, he didn't have asthma. Larry did not see any physician on a regular schedule.

Now, look at Andrew, an eight-year-old boy with asthma. His disease was just as severe as Larry's. A few years ago, Andrew and his family were stuck on the same roller coaster as Larry is now. A family friend recommended an allergist, and they began to work with her. Andrew's mom learned about the chronic nature of asthma. She also learned that there were medications she could give Andrew daily that would just about stop the ups and downs, and she learned to recognize early when things were getting worse for Andrew, taking action right away. The emergency room visits stopped.

What's the difference between Larry and Andrew? Recognizing the nature of the problem. The ability to understand asthma as a chronic problem allowed Andrew and his family to take the necessary steps to begin to control it and then prevent it. Because Larry viewed his asthma as spontaneous or episodic, he saw himself as powerless to prevent it and was left reacting to it whenever problems erupted.

2. PREVENTION (BY AVOIDANCE)

When I think of preventing problems by avoiding them, I can't help but think of an old Henny Youngman (comedian) joke:

> The patient says, "Doctor, it hurts when I do this." The doctor replies, "Then don't do that!"

Okay, I am a sucker for one-liners. But, we know that jokes are funny because they contain some element of the truth.

We live in a world containing dust mites, air pollution, smoke, viruses, animals, and odors, among other irritants. To a person without asthma, these things may be a nuisance, but to the person with asthma, these things can trigger an attack. The key point here is to know your asthma triggers and avoid them when possible, or at least to limit your exposure to them.

Let's look at Larry again. Larry knows that smoky environments really trigger his asthma, but he hangs around with his friends who smoke anyway; he noticed he coughed more around them, but he didn't want to make them angry by asking them to stop. He also loved cologne and didn't want to give it up because he liked it—even though it seemed to make his asthma act up as well. Lastly, Larry had a dog at home and every time he groomed him, Larry started coughing—but he loved his dog and would never dream of giving him up. In fact, he was actually thinking of getting a second one.

What is the result of Larry's behaviors? Because Larry did not avoid his triggers, he had more chronic and persistent asthma symptoms than would otherwise be the case.

How about Andrew? When he first started working with his allergist, Andrew was waking in the middle of the night at least once a month with asthma attacks. The allergist determined that dust mites triggered his symptoms and together with Mom explored what preventive steps could be used to avoid these problems. Understanding that things like strong scents, chemical odors, and perfumes seemed to make Andrew's asthma a little bit worse, Mom stopped wearing perfumes and changed to using non-irritant cleaners.

Andrew's mom also noticed that playing outside on days when the ozone levels were high, he might also have problems, so she made certain that on those days, she'd find other activities for him to do indoors. Because the family was avoiding those things that triggered Andrew's asthma, he had less trouble with acute asthma symptoms and attacks. Again, the roller coaster ride of uncontrolled asthma was derailed.

3. PULMONARY FUNCTION TESTS

Ironically, a person with asthma may report feeling well when in fact their lungs may not be doing well at all. Pulmonary function tests (PFTs) can be used to gather information on a person's current lung function beyond simply asking how the person feels. These tests add objective data to what a person feels. Hopefully, these tests confirm that things are indeed going well; if this is not the case, the treatment plan can be adjusted as needed. Let's look at Larry and Andrew to see how PFTs can be useful.

Larry rarely sees the same doctor twice so his care is fragmented. Pulmonary function tests are never done and problems develop silently until he develops symptoms. Without this additional knowledge, Larry does not have the impetus he needs to stay on top of his asthma. Because he feels well, there is no information to tell him that he should be treating his asthma—when he really should!

Andrew sees his allergist twice a year and his lung function is checked. It is typically found to be normal; this is reassurance that the treatment plan is working.

What's the difference between these examples?

Andrew has evidence that his lung function is good and this serves as reinforcement that the treatment plan is working; Larry, who doesn't have that information, just goes by how he feels. But we know that you can feel good and still have reduced lung function. If you are running around with reduced lung function, you risk any trigger pushing you into a full-blown severe asthma attack.

If Larry knew that his pulmonary function was 30% less than it should be, it would lead to more aggressive treatment; but since he doesn't have that information, he doesn't feel the need to change treatment. This all ties back to understanding the problem—asthma is a chronic illness. It doesn't just go away when there are no external symptoms.

4. PHARMACEUTICALS

The approach here is to recommend the right amount of medicine needed to control asthma, nothing less and nothing more. It's a balancing act. As a physician, I want to prescribe enough medicine to keep someone healthy but not any more than is needed. This helps to minimize side effects and keep the treatment regimen as simple as possible.

When it comes to pharmaceuticals, think of treating asthma as climbing stairs. Treating the mildest form of asthma requires only going up one step. That is, a bronchodilator inhaler or nebulizer is all that is needed. If the asthma is not controlled here, you ascend to the next step—using an inhaled anti-inflammatory medicine or a pill such as Singulair. This step-up approach is repeated until the right combination of medications are found.

A physician's challenge is to identify what kind and how much medicine is right for each person—not too little and not too much.

When Larry had a severe asthma attack, he would only take the medicine prescribed by the doctors for a few days, until he felt better. This is because Larry viewed his asthma as an acute problem that needed only on-the-spot treatment. When he felt better, he thought his asthma had gone away. As a result, Larry didn't take any type of regular asthma medicine other than his bronchodilator, which he used *daily*—a sign that he was stuck in crisis mode. (Remember the Rules of Two.) Larry's therapy stayed at one level—a level below that which he really needed.

How about Andrew? The doctor started Andrew off with a basic bronchodilator inhaler to treat his symptoms. Realizing that the bronchodilator wasn't enough, the doctor stepped up treatment, adding a second medicine taken daily, which worked well.

What's the difference between these examples?

Andrew and his doctor have found out the right amount of medicine and Andrew takes it regularly—even when he feels well. Larry, in contrast, relies only on his bronchodilator, and never steps up to using an inhaled anti-inflammatory inhaler every day; he just goes from one attack to the next.

5. PLAN

You need a plan. If you have asthma, you should always keep your short-acting bronchodilator available. But is that enough? Working with your physician, develop a plan that tells you when to take action; what action(s) to take when you develop coughing, wheezing, and chest tightness; and when to seek help.

Larry's plan is crisis-driven. When he gets sick, his plan is just to increase the number of times he uses his bronchodilator until things either improve or he has to seek emergency help. It's a one-level plan. Clearly, his asthma is in charge here.

In contrast, Andrew's mom knows that if he starts to get a cold (a major trigger for his asthma) and he starts to have a certain cough, there is potential for problems. Following Andrew's asthma action plan, she immediately starts supporting him with more acute treatment (using breathing treatments or his bronchodilator up to four times a day). She understands that if things quickly get better, no further action is needed; if things don't improve or worsen, she calls her allergist and Andrew can be seen in the office earlier in the course of the attack. Andrew's asthma action plan tells Mom what to do and when to do it!

6. PATIENT–PHYSICIAN RELATIONSHIP

A long-term, good relationship with the right kind of doctor is a must!

This book intends to provide you with knowledge and a framework for beating your asthma. Principle 6 is an important part of this effort. Engaging in a collaborative relationship with a physician, built on mutual respect and dialogue, will serve you well. You want to work with someone who listens to you and values your input as part of the treatment team. This may be an allergist or a pediatrician, family physician or internist.

Look at Larry—he's just too busy to see a doctor regularly. What he'll do instead is see whatever physician he can at the nearest Emergency Room or Acute Care clinic. He rarely sees the same physician twice. In these settings, though, physicians are more concerned about treating the acute problems Larry has and getting him over his current attack. Their purpose is not to provide the longer term care he needs to manage his chronic condition; they deal with emergencies, since that's their job. Yet, as good as they are, these facilities may not have the longer term view of the allergist who would say: "Larry, this has happened to you three times in the past three months. What do we need to do to change that?"

In contrast, Andrew and his mom have been seeing the same physician for a few years now. Mom is able to relate Andrew's history to the doctor. The physician listens to her, values her input, and views her as an expert in what is currently happening with Andrew. The physician is then able to bring her expertise to bear on what changes need to be made to Andrew's treatment plan to improve control.

What's the difference between these examples?

Larry doesn't have a long-term relationship with a physician who understands asthma, whereas Andrew and his mom have been seeing the same allergy physician for several years now. Mom has learned to trust the physician and the physician has learned to trust her. Mom is able to communicate when things are happening with Andrew, and the treatment plan can be adjusted based upon that. This is a powerful relationship.

7. POSITIVE MINDSET

The seventh principle may seem softer but it is no less important: maintaining a positive mindset.

We are not talking about managing or beating asthma simply by having a positive or optimistic attitude. At this point in time, we have no research proving that this can be done. The positive mindset I describe here has more to do with several psychological characteristics that appear to me to make it easier for a person to remain adherent to the treatment plan.

I want to avoid what Dr. Jimmie Holland has called the tyranny of optimism in her book, *The Human Side of Cancer*. During her long career as a psychiatrist at Sloan-Kettering Memorial Cancer Center in New York, Dr. Holland has observed a multitude of coping styles in people afflicted with cancer. She has discredited the popular viewpoint that optimism is the only feasible coping mechanism for these patients. I completely agree with her. We all have unique coping styles and these are difficult to change. Some of us are naturally more pessimistic, others more optimistic. It would be silly of me to push a mom to be optimistic when she has been awake half the night with a coughing, wheezing child ending up in the Emergency Room at 5 AM, and is now late for work, with her husband away on a business trip. I might get a tongue-lashing or worse—and I would most certainly deserve it!

Having said this, the positive mindset is still very useful. "Positive mindset" in this context is composed of optimism, ownership, and something the field of positive psychology calls *grit* (passion and perseverance). Having the optimistic mindset needed to overcome asthma is about having a hopeful attitude that helps you stay engaged in your treatment. Staying engaged is important because when you have a persistent disease, it requires persistence of effort on your part. This persistence is sometimes necessary to overcome denial and allows you to take ownership of your asthma. This allows you to maintain the positive actions needed in controlling asthma successfully over time.

Poor Larry. He believes he is a victim of his asthma. This prevents him from taking responsibility for his illness. He sees it as something that's happening to him and seems unable to see the importance of his role in treatment. He has yet to learn that there are certain things he can do to prevent many of his attacks from even happening. Although he has prescribed medicines, he may take them only until he feels better and then stops. In other words, he seems to have little or no persistence and perseverance when it comes to the effort required of him to really treat his asthma. He views his asthma from the mindset of a victim, leaving him feeling somewhat hopeless and helpless. This is a sad state indeed.

Alternately, Andrew's mom thinks about his asthma regularly and never puts it out of her mind completely. Andrew's mom also understands that it's she and Andrew who are responsible for dealing with problems as, or even before, they arise (they "own" the asthma) and that there are things she can do to make sure the asthma doesn't get out of control. She has an optimistic outlook, and Andrew has learned to adopt the same attitude. As a result, she and Andrew are not victims; they are empowered. They have a positive mindset—an outlook that says "we can deal with everything as it arises"—that leads them to stay engaged and in control of Andrew's asthma.

What's the difference between Larry and Andrew?

Larry doesn't understand. He has a responsibility to do certain things to help himself and to really follow the other six principles we talked about already, but he does not see this. As a result, he stays stuck in a helpless, victim mentality.

Andrew's mom understands that his asthma is treatable (she has an optimistic outlook) so she focuses on what the family needs to do (they take ownership) and keeps an eye on Andrew's needs and treatment over time (persistence) to ensure the illness stays under control.

By persisting in your efforts, you create a positive mindset and sense of control. This leads to better asthma control and because your asthma is under better control, you will have a more positive mindset. It's a reinforcing cycle that will help you to ultimately beat asthma!

We have certainly covered a lot of information in this chapter, and hopefully it is now clear that better outcomes for asthma are possible. Seeing an allergist will help to ensure that you have the best chance of controlling your asthma. That being said, it is unlikely that all asthmatics will see an allergist, so I am writing this book to help you be the best you can be, no matter which physician you partner with.

When I see someone who is beating their asthma—I see that this person is able to:

1. recognize that asthma is a chronic illness that must be continually managed (they understand the problem)
2. know the things they need to avoid (prevention)
3. obtain objective data on their lung functioning (have regular pulmonary function tests)
4. have and follow their asthma action plan
5. use medications as prescribed
6. work with a competent doctor who listens and wants them to be active contributors to their treatment plan

7. remain positive in spite of challenges and setbacks, taking ownership of their role in managing asthma and persisting with treatment to maintain control of the disease.

These seven principles are the framework aimed at *beating asthma*. So, let's move on, where we will spend a chapter on each of the seven principles, building on this foundation. Each chapter will better prepare you to take control of your asthma and to get back to the life you really want to live!

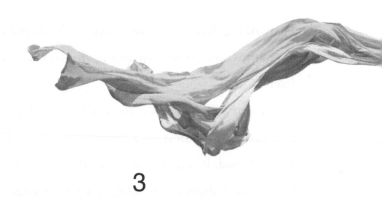

3

Understanding the Problem

To some people, asthma is a disease associated with weakness. Nothing could be further from the truth.

Down through the ages, many notable, powerful people have been afflicted with asthma. Among them are five U.S. presidents: Van Buren, Coolidge, Kennedy, Theodore Roosevelt, and Wilson. In addition, Ludwig van Beethoven, Peter the Great, Charles Dickens, and Alice Cooper, as well as world-class athlete Jerome Bettis (NFL) and Olympic Gold Medalists Nancy Hogshead and Jackie Joyner-Kersee, all had asthma, yet all are or were exceptional people in their own right.

Asthmatics come from all races, all walks of life, and all professions. They are rich, poor, young, and old. I have taken care of big, hairy, imposing men with asthma as well as the most vulnerable, innocent young children. Asthma does not discriminate.

Why point this out here? To remind you that asthma is not a disease of weakness or a mental disease. Asthma is a lung issue. Period. It is not a disease of the mind. As with any chronic illness, asthma can be *affected* by what goes on in our minds (such as stress), but it is lung disease.

In this chapter, we will look at the way the lungs function in individuals with asthma. By doing this, we will lay a strong foundation for understanding how to treat asthma.

The first important point to remember is this: Asthma is a *chronic* disease with periods of acute worsening. It is always present, even if you are not currently experiencing problems. This is a point that may not be clear to people who believe that asthma is present only when it is causing breathing problems.

Some of my colleagues have compared asthma to an iceberg. The small piece of the iceberg that sits above the water is like the symptoms of asthma that you can see. Just like an iceberg, however, there is a much larger part that sits unseen below the surface. As it was with the Titanic and its encounter with an iceberg, it is this hidden part of asthma that can cause big problems. It is the part below the surface that gets you in real trouble.

WHAT CAUSES ASTHMA? MUSCLES, MUCUS, AND INFLAMMATION, OH MY!

The simplest way to define asthma is this: Asthma is *reversible* airway obstruction. In other words, blockage (obstruction) occurs in the lungs, and this blockage can be reversed. This is different from a lung disease called COPD (chronic obstructive lung disease), in which the lung structure has been permanently changed (most often due to tobacco use).

What are the airways? In the past, you may have seen the lungs portrayed as air-filled balloons, but this oversimplifies things greatly. An upside-down tree is a more accurate representation, in which the thick trunk of the tree subdivides into many branches, with the branches becoming smaller and smaller in size. On the smallest branches are the leaves.

In the lungs, the trachea or windpipe is like the tree trunk because it is the largest airway. The trachea then subdivides into branches that continue to subdivide over and over into thousands of smaller and smaller branches, until we arrive at the smallest unit in the lungs, the alveoli, which are like the leaves on the tree. (The alveoli are where oxygen is taken into the bloodstream and carbon dioxide is removed.) All of these tubes, branches, and alveoli together are called the airways. It is in these many branches where the reversible obstruction occurs.

What causes the obstruction or blockage? Three key things happen:

1. Muscles in the walls of the airways tighten.

2. The airway wall becomes inflamed.

3. The airways produce increased mucus.

Let's look more in depth at each of these three issues.

First, let's look at the muscles that tighten. The airway walls are made up in part by a type of muscle called smooth muscle. Unlike the muscles in your arms or legs, this smooth muscle is *not* under voluntary control. But, just like other muscles, it can contract and relax. When someone has asthma, the muscle tissue is twitchy or hyper-reactive; it responds to irritation more quickly and to an exaggerated degree than in non-asthmatic lungs. When this smooth muscle contracts, it tightens and narrows the airways.

Now, picture this process happening in thousands of airways at the same time. The lumens, or spaces within the airways, become narrow, and this makes it much harder for air to get through. In other words, there is increased resistance to the flow of air. Because of this, feelings of chest tightness or shortness of breath, as well as cough and wheezing, may occur. This muscle tightening makes it hard to breathe.

You can demonstrate for yourself what happens here by a simple experiment using a plastic straw. Puff air through the straw and feel how easily it flows through. Now, repeat this, but pinch the straw between your thumb and forefinger. Notice how it becomes harder to move the air through the straw. Go ahead and pinch the straw in two different places. It becomes even more difficult to move air through. Imagine this happening in many locations in the thousands of airways that make up the lungs, and you can understand what an important role this muscle tightening plays in causing symptoms. In the past, it was thought that this was the only problem with the lungs in asthma. We now know the problem is a bit more complicated.

Secondly, inflammation occurs in the lungs. A complex reaction takes place in the airways of a person with asthma during an attack. The body makes chemical products that are released into the lungs. These chemicals, called mediators, summon or draw white blood cells into the walls of the airways. These white blood cells normally help us fight off infection. Their accumulation here in the lungs in asthma, however, wreaks havoc. The airway walls become thicker and less flexible, the spaces within the airways become even more narrow, and the airways become stiffer. As a result, it's more difficult for air to flow through them.

Most of us at some time have experienced inflammation in our bodies. A good example would be what oftentimes occurs following a bee sting or insect bite. The area may swell immediately, and, in some cases, the swelling may last for several days. Chemical mediators are released and white blood cells are called into the area where the sting occurred. This area also becomes red and puffy, with the skin here not as soft as the surrounding unaffected skin. This area is inflamed! Now, imagine inflammation happening across all the airways in the lungs. Once it occurs, this inflammation may take *months* to completely resolve!

Lastly, the asthmatic lung has a problem with mucus. All lungs, even healthy lungs, produce mucus; it is part of an intricate defense system that maintains health. This mucus moves up from the smaller airways to the larger airways. It can trap airborne particles that might cause damage to the body and moves them up and out of the lungs.

People with asthma, especially during an attack, produce more mucus in their airways than usual. This mucus is thicker and more difficult to move out of the lungs. It builds up in the spaces of the airways and adds to the obstruction together with the muscle tightening and inflammation.

As an example, think about what happens when a drain blocks up in your home. When the pipes are new and clean inside, water drains easily. As time passes, gunk becomes stuck to the inside of the drainpipes. It may be a combination of grease, hair, and who knows what! As this happens, the flow of water down the drain becomes slower and slower until it becomes blocked. Then, of course, it's time to call the plumber to clean the mess out of the pipes. So, think of all this mucus as sort of *gumming up* the airways.

Now, how do these three pieces fit together? Normally, air flows in and out of the lungs with relative ease. As a result, oxygen is taken into the bloodstream and carbon dioxide is removed. When airway muscles tighten, increased mucus is produced, and inflammation occurs. This results in partial or complete blockage of many of the smaller airways. As a result, air has a hard time getting to where it needs to be. Some of the airways trap air in and some do not receive air at all. This is why, very quickly, the amount of oxygen that gets into the person's bloodstream falls. This is seen very early on in an asthma attack.

Also in the early stages of an asthma attack, lung obstruction causes the person to breathe more rapidly, and the amount of carbon dioxide in the blood is reduced. As things worsen, the amount of carbon dioxide then rises, because it can't escape the lungs. When this occurs, immediate life-saving action must be taken. It means that the lungs are not able to keep up with the demands of the body. They are failing. Usually, at this point, the person must be helped to breathe using a machine called a ventilator.

Thankfully, when we consider all the asthma attacks that occur each year, this scenario is relatively rare. It does demonstrate, though, just how bad things can get during a severe asthma episode.

As we will see later in the book, this whole process can be triggered by allergens (animal dander and pollens) in which case it is known as *allergic asthma*, or by irritants (smoke and air pollution), called *non-allergic asthma*. Often, it is a combination of both allergic and non-allergic factors that trigger asthma.

To sum it up, muscles surrounding the airway walls become twitchy and tighten, inflammation takes place, and more mucus is produced in the airways. All of this adds up to produce the signs and symptoms of asthma, including cough, shortness of breath, wheezing, and the production of thick mucus. These things make it hard to breathe.

How does this understanding affect how we treat asthma?

Well, visualizing the lungs as a tree you can see why it takes time for medicine to get into all those nooks and crannies. Once you have an asthma attack, it may take months for the lungs to return to normal, simply because there is so much surface area involved that needs to heal.

Understanding the problem of asthma will thus help you to set more realistic expectations for full recovery because you will recognize that recovery takes time. This will also help you be more hopeful because you won't misinterpret a time-intensive recovery as poor progress. In an era when most things move at the speed of light, from instant messaging to streaming video, it helps to remember that some things can't be delivered on-demand; there is simply no replacement for time and correct treatment when it comes to controlling your asthma.

Let's move on to the next principle—the cornerstone of asthma treatment—prevention.

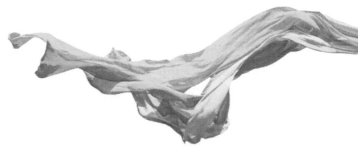

4

Prevention by Avoidance: Mites, Pollens, and Molds

As Benjamin Franklin once wisely said, "An ounce of prevention is worth a pound of cure." Arguably, nowhere else is the idea of prevention by avoidance more important and useful than when managing your asthma.

If we are aware of those things that can make asthma worse (asthma triggers), then avoiding these triggers becomes the cornerstone of asthma treatment—not drugs, not meditation, not some secret potion or alternative technique known to but a few.

It is the prevention of asthma attacks by the avoidance of asthma triggers that is our focus in this chapter and the next. This may all just seem like common sense to you, and I would agree with that, but, in our quest for asthma control, we cannot afford to let this stone go unturned. So, let's examine this whole area of prevention by avoidance.

Why is prevention by avoidance important? Once you are exposed to an asthma trigger, a whole series of complex events takes place in the lungs (muscles, mucus, and inflammation, oh my!) If we prevent these reactions from occurring in the first place, we can stop the asthma events that follow.

Asthma triggers can cause problems directly in the lungs, or, by first causing a reaction in the nose. In fact, 75% of children with asthma have allergies. Avoiding asthma triggers, whether allergic or non-allergic, helps keep the nose in a healthy state, reducing problems with asthma. We aren't exactly certain as to why this is true, but the connection between what happens in the nose and then follows in the lungs is real. Avoiding known asthma triggers can reduce the number of asthma attacks and improve lung function, reducing the intensity of treatment needed.

Asthma triggers are many and varied. For our review, I have divided them into three categories: allergic, non-allergic, and other. In this chapter, we will look at the allergic triggers.

ALLERGIC TRIGGERS

Allergic triggers are a two-way street. Allergens have the effects that they do when:

1. the specific allergens themselves are present in your environment, and

2. your body makes allergy antibodies and responds to the allergens.

It is the combination of allergy in you, plus exposure to the things you are allergic to that triggers a reaction. If either the allergen is not present, or you are not allergic to it, no reaction occurs. The most common allergic triggers for asthma include house dust mites, animal dander, pollens, and molds. Let's look at each of these allergens in more detail and explore some ways in which you might avoid them.

House dust mites. Dust mites are microscopic little critters that are found in common household items like carpeting, upholstered furniture, and bedding (pillows, mattress, and box springs). Dust mites do not bite or carry disease, but they do consume shed human skin cells, producing fecal pellets along the way. It is actually their fecal pellets in house dust that we are allergic to. (Okay, am I telling you too much now? Ugh!)

Dust mites are not found where the humidity is very low (in the desert, or at high altitudes), but they are found in just about every American home. So, if these mites are found just about everywhere, how on earth can we avoid them? Is it a lost cause? Not at all. The following are steps you can easily take to reduce your exposure to dust mites.

- *Cover mattress and pillows with allergy covers.* These covers trap the mite allergen inside and don't allow it to get out. The best products to use are those made of tightly woven fabrics, which will prevent the migration of dust mite allergens through the covering.[1]

- *Do not have carpeting in the home, at least not in the bedroom.* I encourage you to make your bedroom an allergen-free zone as much as possible. If you are spending eight hours daily there, having reduced exposure to your triggers for that period of time can be very helpful. You can't successfully vacuum all the mite allergen out of fabrics or carpets. Control what you can as best as you can.

- *Launder pillow covers and sheets once a week in* hot *water.* Many of us may have gotten used to cold-water washing, but that doesn't really inactivate dust mite allergens.

- As far as furniture type, *leather or vinyl furniture is better than upholstered.* Because these materials can be wiped down, surface dust can be removed. Dust mites really love to live in fabrics with lots of nooks and crannies.

- *Reduce the use of ceiling fans* so you don't keep house dust suspended in the air. Using a ceiling fan, stirring up air currents in the room, will pick up mite allergens and suspend them in the air and you will inhale them. If the air in the room settles down, the dust mite allergens will fall to surfaces within twenty minutes or so.

For a person with asthma, what can't be seen *can* hurt them. Dust mites fall into this category. Making small changes in how you make your bed, launder sheets, and cool and furnish your home can go a long way to help diminish dust-related asthma triggers.

Animal dander. Clearly, Americans have a love affair with cats and dogs. There are 93.6 million pet cats in America (33% of households with at least one cat), and 77 million dogs (39% of households have at least one dog).[2] Chances are very high that even if you don't own a pet, you are friends with someone who does. There is a high probability of being exposed to some type of animal dander. If you are allergic to these animals, your symptoms can be triggered by this exposure.

As an example, let me relate a story told to me by Dr. David Meadows, an outstanding allergy physician. It seems that there was a young boy under his care with significant allergies and asthma. Overall, he was well controlled. At one time he started to have problems with acute nasal allergy and asthma symptoms—but only when he went to school, and only in the morning!

With some great medical detective work, David found that this child was sitting next to a classmate who owned a horse. She would groom her horse every morning before coming to school. The young boy was highly allergic to horse dander. His problems were triggered by being exposed to horse allergen carried on the clothing of his classmate! The problem was resolved by simply having him change seats in the class. You don't even have to own an animal to be exposed to and to have your asthma triggered by animal dander!

So, what are you to do if animals trigger your asthma?

- The gold standard of asthma treatment is this: *If you have allergic asthma due to certain animals, do not have these animals in your home.* They must be avoided. The more severe your sensitivity, the more important it is to adhere to this standard. Anything less will expose you to the risk of ongoing problems with uncontrolled asthma.

- *Avoid prolonged exposure to animals you are allergic to in other settings, such as in the homes of friends or family.* If friends have pets and tell you that they will keep them out of sight and away while you are visiting, this is usually not enough to prevent exposure, since the stuff you are allergic to is found in the carpets, in dust, and even on the walls.

- It is important to remember that *if you have a pet in the home for some time and then remove it, it may take up to a year for that allergen to fall to levels in a home without pets.* Animal dander lasts a long time, even after cleaning. Usually, you have to do more vigorous cleaning, including the walls and fixtures, to begin the process of returning your home to a non-dander zone.

As an allergist I've learned that it can be a big battle to convince people to remove their pets from the home, because animals become part of the family. It's tough because of the emotional attachment we have to them.

To break the tension on this subject, I sometimes joke with my patients that they don't have to get rid of the cat or dog. Instead, just let them live in the house, and you can move outside. Of course, I have yet to see anyone follow this advice!

For those patients who absolutely cannot imagine saying goodbye to a pet, I focus on using increasing levels of avoidance. That is,

- keep the animal outside of the home
- if the animals are inside the home, limit them to one area of the house
- keep the animal out of the bedroom.

The use of an air filter known as a HEPA filter may be of some use here as well. These are freestanding units that filter out animal dander and other allergens. They may be used in the bedroom as well as throughout the home. The size of the unit should be matched to the size of the room in which it will be used.

Other measures to reduce animal dander have been recommended, including bathing the pets frequently, using wipes to remove the allergen, and frequent grooming, but it is not certain that these activities really will make a difference in the overall amount of allergen you are exposed to.

There are no particular breeds of animals that are truly hypoallergenic. Yet, one recent development has been the breeding of naturally occurring mutant cats and dogs that produce little to none of the major allergens!

Allerca is a company doing this for five years now. This is a consideration for those who want to have a cat or dog but who are allergic. As with any new scientific development, however, it comes with a price tag. As of April 2011, the price for one of these animals ranged from about $7,000 to $23,000. It is still no guarantee that you will not be affected by a more minor allergen. If interested, you can look into this and decide for yourself whether it is worth the cost!*

Pollens. Along with dust mites and animal dander, those with allergic asthma also have to consider the possible effects of pollens from trees, grasses, and weeds. These pollens, which are spread on wind currents and can travel long distances, can

---

* http://www.allerca.com/index.html

cause symptoms in both asthma and nasal allergies. These tiny pollen particles are inhaled, and, if you are allergic to them, they produce symptoms. Pollen can do this directly in the lungs or by producing problems in the nose, affecting the lungs indirectly.

In general, there are fairly distinct pollen seasons, with trees pollinating in the early spring, grasses in the later spring, and weeds in the fall. There are regional variations and unique species that cause this schedule to vary. In Texas, for example, we have a tree known as mountain cedar (a juniper tree), which pollinates from November to February or March. Our other trees typically begin to pollinate in February, and grasses in late March or early April, causing problems from then right through the fall. As a result, here in Texas, our pollen seasons begin earlier and may last longer than in the more northern parts of the country. (Lucky us!) Your local allergist should have a good understanding of how these seasons are structured where you live. The website pollen.com is a useful source of information as well.

So, given the fact that these pollens are found pretty much everywhere and may travel over some distance to reach us, how in the world can we prevent problems by avoiding them?

Here are some tips that may be useful:

- Avoid extended outdoor activity during the pollen seasons, especially when winds are high.
- Take your medications.

- Keep windows closed during pollen season, especially during the day (home and auto!)
- Use the air conditioner in your vehicle.
- Stay inside during mid-day and afternoon hours, when pollen counts are highest.
- Take a shower, wash your hair, and change clothing after working or playing outdoors.[3]

If you follow these few tips, you will be taking important actions to prevent asthma problems due to pollen triggers.

MOLDS

Mold and fungi are a part of the natural decay process of organic materials, such as leaves, grass, and other plants. As with pollens, they are spread by wind currents. They tend to be more abundant in areas with high humidity and can also be found in structures that have undergone some type of water damage or flooding. When such damage or flooding occurs, it is important that mold remediation be part of the rebuilding process. A dilute solution of household bleach and water is very effective at removing mold. The Centers for Disease Control (http://www.cdc.gov/mold/faqs.htm) and the American College of Allergy, Asthma and Immunology (http://www.acaai.org) both have some helpful information on molds, mold prevention, and mold remediation on their websites.

The helpful measures for mold avoidance are similar to those for pollen avoidance:

- Avoid extended outdoor activity when the mold count is high, especially when winds are strong.[*]
- Take your medications. This is extremely important because those asthmatics who are allergic to one mold called alternaria may be at risk of more severe asthma attacks.
- Avoid mowing the lawn or raking leaves. If you must, then wear a good protective mask while doing so.
- Keep windows closed during times of high mold counts.

Although a lot of the information we just reviewed may be common sense, it is important to pay attention to the details of allergen avoidance in your efforts to beat asthma.

On to the next chapter, where we will look at prevention as it relates to irritants (non-allergens), as well as other triggers such as exercise, reflux (heartburn), and sinus infections.

---

[*] Another good source for pollen and mold spore counts can be found at www. aaaai.org/global/nab-pollen-counts.aspx

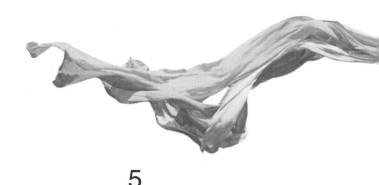

5

Prevention by Avoidance: Non-Allergic Triggers

While allergic triggers only cause problems for people who are allergic to them, non-allergic triggers can be called *equal opportunity offenders*. What do I mean by this?

When you are allergic, it is like having the key that turns the switch that starts the engine of asthmatic inflammation. No key (no allergy), no inflammation.

With non-allergic triggers (especially the *irritants* listed below), no key is necessary. The irritant itself pushes a start button that turns the engine on directly. In short, if you have asthma, any of the triggers listed in this chapter can harm or affect you. You need not be allergic.

IRRITANTS

Chemical odors. Many people with asthma cannot use cleaning agents with strong odors without triggering their asthma. Using lower irritant cleaners or delegating the task to someone else if possible (now that's a side benefit!) are the two means of avoiding these potent triggers.

There are some individuals, however, who work in jobs and industries where the exposure to chemicals happens often. Certain chemicals in the workplace produce *occupational asthma*. Here it is not just the irritant effect at work but a complex inflammatory reaction that takes place in the lungs.

Symptoms associated with occupational asthma are worse when you are at work, and better when you're away from it. If you discover a connection between worsening asthma and chemicals used in your job, you will need to either use a specialized breathing protection device (i.e., a respirator) in the workplace, or you may actually have to change jobs to prevent serious long-term health problems. The OSHA website has good information on occupational asthma if you need to learn more.[*]

Perfumes and scents. Asthma can be triggered by breathing in the fumes that these substances give off.

This is not just perfumes or colognes that you spray or daub on your body. Also included are the scents that may

---

[*] www.osha.gov/SLTC/occupationalasthma/index.html

accompany the detergents, soaps, and lotions that you use to care for your skin or clothes. Unscented versions of these products are plentiful in the marketplace, and they are worth seeking out to ensure that you don't unintentionally trigger your asthma.

Of course, sometimes you may end up on the elevator with someone drenched in perfume or cologne (sort of a sneak attack, if you will). The best approach here is to quickly put as much clean air space between you and the offending agent as you can. This may mean stepping to a new spot in the elevator or exiting the elevator on the next floor.

Smoke. Tobacco smoke and asthma do not mix and simply have to be kept apart. If you have asthma, you absolutely should not smoke. Similarly, if you live with a smoker, that person should smoke outside the home, and never while riding in your vehicle. Neither rolling down a car window nor cracking open the back door of the house while someone is smoking is going to do the trick.

Other potential sources of smoke exposure include campfires, wildfires, and fireplaces, as well as some bars and restaurants (secondhand smoke), although over time fewer and fewer commercial establishments are allowing smoking indoors.

Air pollution. Here in Texas, especially in the summertime when the air is hot and there is very little wind, we have elevated ozone levels in the air. Unfortunately, this phenomenon is not limited to Texas: elevated ozone levels can be seen in many parts of the nation, especially in urban areas.

Ozone, a gas that cannot be seen or smelled, is a respiratory tract irritant, even to people without asthma. For convenience, the government grades ozone levels from green to yellow, orange, and red, where green represents the lowest level, and red, the highest level.

Ozone levels seem to be at their highest levels during traffic rush hour in the late afternoon and early evening. If you have asthma, ozone levels above green—especially above yellow—require your attention. During these times, outdoor physical activity should be limited. In addition, keeping windows in your home and vehicle closed with air vents closed or on recirculate should help. Ozone levels and alerts are readily available and are typically part of the weather forecast on local radio and television stations. One of the EPA websites is a good resource as well.*

Interestingly, ozone gets the most press, but it is only one of many components of air pollution that can produce problems. Others include sulfur dioxide and diesel exhaust particles. The total Air Quality Index (which takes into account not just ozone but these other pollutants as well) ranges from green (safe) to maroon (hazardous). Staying aware of this daily

---

* http://www.airnow.gov/ for information on current pollution levels and more

reading can guide your decision on whether to go outdoors or stay inside on any given day.

MEDICATIONS

Aspirin/NSAIDS. Some people have asthma triggered by aspirin or aspirin-like drugs such as ibuprofen or naproxen. This class of drugs is known as NSAIDs (for non-steroidal anti-inflammatory drugs).

I once had a patient who had a severe asthma attack two hours after taking ibuprofen and who ended up in the ICU. This happened on two different occasions! Both times, a well-meaning relative gave the medication to her. These drugs clearly can cause serious problems.

NSAIDs are more likely to be a problem as a trigger if you have nasal polyps and chronic sinusitis with asthma. In general, I have my asthma patients—even those without nasal polyps and chronic sinusitis but who have had problems with aspirin in the past—avoid NSAIDs. For most people with asthma and NSAID sensitivity, acetaminophen is a safe alternative medicine to treat pain. It is best to discuss this issue with your personal physician.

In some cases, aspirin is absolutely required as a medication. In such situations, a procedure known as oral desensitization can be successfully accomplished under the guidance of an allergist. Oral desensitization is the graded ingestion of aspirin, beginning with extremely low doses and progressing to higher and higher doses, until one reaches the standard dose, which he or she must remain on without interruption every day to remain desensitized. As one might expect, this procedure does have its risks, and allergic reactions can be seen as the dose is raised during the process.

Beta-Blockers. These medications are frequently used in the treatment of heart disease, hypertension, migraine headaches, and glaucoma (eye drops). They work by blocking a cell receptor known as the beta-receptor. If asthma worsens after beginning these types of medicines, an alternative drug needs to be used.

OTHER SITUATIONS

Gastro-esophageal Reflux (GERD). In some patients, asthma is triggered by gastro-esophageal reflux (GERD), sometimes just called reflux or heartburn. Reflux can irritate the lungs directly or cause nasal disease and sinusitis that worsen asthma.

Most times, GERD is accompanied by symptoms such as heartburn, but not always. Many physicians will treat asthma patients with difficult to control asthma using a month or more of anti-reflux medications just on suspicion that GERD may be causing problems.

Most cases cannot be simply cured by avoidance of certain foods. In severe cases surgery may be necessary.

Sinusitis. Sinusitis, a bacterial infection of the sinuses is a common complicating factor for asthmatics. Sinusitis is treated with antibiotics. Often brought about by any of the triggers we looked at previously (e.g., animal and other allergies, smoke, and strong odors), it can often be prevented by using the avoidance measures we discussed. The use of some form of nasal wash with saline may help as a natural, non-medication method to treat or prevent sinusitis. In the long term, usually medications—and sometimes allergy shots—may be needed to successfully treat the allergies that can lead to recurrent sinus infections.

Lastly, one important consideration is to get the influenza vaccination every fall. Influenza infection can cause major asthma problems; immunization reduces the risk.

Pregnancy. While it is in the strictest sense not an asthma trigger, I wanted to take a few moments to discuss asthma and pregnancy.

In two-thirds of pregnancies, asthma stays at the same level or improves, but in one-third of women, it worsens.

For pregnant women with asthma, the biggest risk to the unborn baby is *not the medications* needed to control it but from *uncontrolled asthma itself.*

The most recent guidelines involving the treatment of asthma in pregnancy, published by the American College of

Obstetrics and Gynecology (ACOG), provide state-of-the-art recommendations.* An obstetrician and allergist working together as a team is the best way to maximize control of the mom's asthma and minimize risk to the unborn baby.

Exercise and asthma. Vigorous exertion will produce symptoms in many people with asthma. This is often referred to as exercise-induced bronchospasm or EIB for short. Asthma symptoms commonly begin 6-8 minutes into a vigorous workout. Typically, the symptoms stop with cessation of exertion and administration of medications.

So, is my recommendation to avoid any type of physical exertion in people with asthma and EIB?

Certainly not!

History is full of stories of elite athletes with asthma who successfully competed in their sport (as noted in an earlier chapter). Often, the onset of EIB symptoms can be prevented by the use of a bronchodilator inhaler 15-30 minutes before physical exertion. If you also use other medications for asthma, it is very important that you take them as directed to help prevent problems with EIB.

The times I do recommend avoiding vigorous exertion for asthmatics is when they are already fighting some type of illness or asthma flare-up, or when outdoor pollution levels

---

* http://emedicine.medscape.com/article/796274-overview

are elevated. Exercising here may make problems worse and recovery may take longer.

There are many non-allergic factors that can trigger asthma. Here, as with the allergic factors, the most potent means of preventing problems is by following a path of strict avoidance. Recalling Ben Franklin's sage advice at the beginning of Chapter 4 and crossing it with a bit of Jerry Lee Lewis, we can say it is quite true that, *a little bit of avoidance practiced well is better than a whole lot of treatment goin' on!*

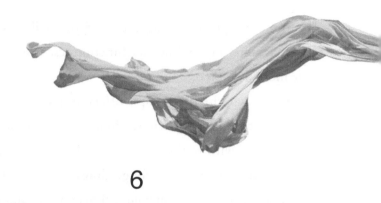

6

Pulmonary Function Tests

When I think about the pulmonary function test, which is one more tool in the asthma-control toolbox, I am reminded of the old tale where three blind men are asked to feel an elephant and guess what it actually is. The first, who touches the elephant's tail, proclaims that it's a snake. The second, who touches the elephant's sturdy side asserts that it's a wall. And the third, who touches the elephant's tusk exclaims that it's a spear. It is none of these things, of course, but instead one of the world's largest living creatures!

Asthma treatment is not so unlike an elephant, with its many different parts that together add up to make an effective whole. Focus on just one part of the treatment and you won't have nearly good enough results. But consider each one important and put them together, and you will become able to beat asthma. The pulmonary function test (PFT) is one of these individual pieces.

On its own, the PFT simply offers insight into whether a person is actually experiencing asthma and, if so, how severely; when placed within the context of the 7-P principles, it becomes a fundamental tool for guiding treatment. One of the best ways to keep control of your asthma is to maintain a good understanding of how your lungs are functioning on a given day or in a certain time period. With this understanding comes the knowledge needed to make wise choices about how to most effectively treat your asthma. Instead of getting blindsided by a surprise asthma attack, you can use your understanding of your current lung function to stay ahead of the game.

Checking in with your physical symptoms is one way to get a read on your asthma status, but as we learned in Chapter 2, individuals are not always aware of what's really going on with their lung function by simply paying attention to how they feel in their bodies.

Pulmonary function tests, and a few others, are designed to help you stay informed of your current lung condition by providing objective measurements (as opposed to subjective measurements, like "I'm feeling fine" or "I think my asthma is acting up.") As you might guess, your doctor is there to let you know when these tests should be administered and how best to use and evaluate them.

When it comes to using tests to stay informed on the state of your asthma, think of other chronic illnesses with which you may be familiar.

- If you have diabetes, you will need to monitor your blood sugar, and your doctor will measure your serum glucose levels.
- If you have high blood pressure, you will need to get regular blood pressure checks.
- If you have cholesterol problems, your doctor will regularly measure your blood lipid levels.

Similarly, if you have asthma, you should regularly monitor how your lungs are doing. Such measurement is commonly done using:

- *pulmonary function tests* (done by your physician)
- *peak flow meter measurements* (done by you).

Several other tests that may be used, although not as commonly, include:

- *pulse oximeter*, a small device that typically clips on your fingertip and indirectly reads the amount of oxygen in your blood. This is most commonly used during an asthma attack or exacerbation.
- *exhaled nitric oxide measurement*, which measures the amount of a gas known as nitric oxide in your exhaled breath. This level gives an idea of how

much inflammation is present in your lungs at that
point in time.

- *blood gases* (or ABG's), which measure the levels of
  oxygen and carbon dioxide in your blood. This test
  is most commonly used in a hospitalized person who
  is severely ill with asthma or other lung problems.
  Because it is not commonly used in outpatient
  asthma care, we will not discuss it further.

Now, let's look at these tests in more detail.

PULMONARY FUNCTION TESTS (PFT)

The PFT provides an objective report on how your
lungs are currently doing. If properly done, the PFT provides
numbers that are a true reflection of your lung function, as
compared to subjective data such as answering a question like,
"How are you feeling?" The PFT is often used initially to help
confirm the diagnosis of asthma and after that to keep track of
your asthma over time.

When you do the PFT, you will be asked to take a really
deep breath in and blow it out as hard, fast and long as you
can. During this time, the test measures two things: how
much total air you are able to blow out of your lungs over 5-7
seconds (this is called FVC or forced vital capacity) and how
fast you are able to exhale that air (FEV1 or forced expiratory
volume at 1 second).

In a person with normal lungs, the majority of air is exhaled within the first second; in a person with asthma it takes longer for the air to come out due to the airway obstruction.

It's like the difference between an air-filled balloon that releases all of its air quickly when you completely let go of it versus the more slow escape of air when you keep the opening pinched and just let a little air out at a time. The pinch-hold of the fingers on the balloon is like the obstruction that is occurring in the airways in asthma.

The numbers returned by the PFT show how much obstruction is happening in the lungs, indicating how healthy or blocked your lungs are.

Sometimes your doctor will administer the PFT once before and once after you have taken an inhaled bronchodilator medicine. This tells how much of the obstruction is easily reversible. These test results, along with the symptoms you describe, will help define the diagnosis of asthma.[*]

If the obstruction is reversible, it's consistent with the diagnosis of asthma and leads us down that treatment path. If the obstruction is not reversible with one breathing treatment, either it is asthma and there is too much obstruction present to quickly reverse it, or it is not asthma, and the obstruction is due to some other condition.

---

[*] Note that if the PFT reveals that the lung obstruction is irreversible, it suggests that there is some kind of fixed problem in the lungs (such as emphysema) and that the person would do best to see a pulmonologist to be evaluated and treated.

There are still a significant number of doctors who do not conduct PFTs in their offices. I can't honestly say whether this reluctance is because of high equipment costs or training and time required to do the test. Regardless, it is a test well within the capabilities of any good physician and staff. When it comes to effective asthma treatment, the PFT is a must.

Current recommendations are that the PFT be done about every 1–2 years on a well-controlled asthma patient and usually more often (every 6 months or less) in more severe asthma patients, whose lung function may change more rapidly.

For those with milder asthma, you might ask, "Why bother with the PFT? Isn't this just driving up the cost of healthcare?"

As we discussed earlier, these tests provide a more complete picture of your lung health than self-reporting alone. In the long run, this will reduce overall cost because it prevents the need for more expensive intervention further down the line.

For example, the Doctor asks, "How are you feeling?" Patient: "Fine." But the PFT shows that the person's lung function is reduced by 30% from normal! The PFT then alerts the physician to look more closely at what is happening with the person's asthma. This often leads to information not previously shared, such as, "I have been waking up at night coughing. Doesn't everyone do that?" or "I have been needing to use my inhaler every day recently."

A person can feel well even when he or she doesn't have normal lung function. The PFT helps you dig a little deeper, identifying problems where they exist. When problems are found, they can be handled with treatment earlier, rather than waiting for problems to worsen significantly.

When your asthma is well controlled, your PFT will be normal.

Now let's move on to a tool that will help you understand how your lung function is from day-to-day.

PEAK FLOW METER

For those asthma patients who would benefit from more regular monitoring of their lung function, there is a simple tool called the peak flow meter. Although the information from the peak flow meter is a bit less precise than the PFT, it is convenient because it's a tiny little instrument that you can hold in your hand and use pretty much anywhere. Simple to perform, the peak flow test involves taking a very deep breath and blowing it out as hard as you can into the device; the result is a number that reflects your lung function right on the spot.

When you first start using your peak flow meter, the goal will be to gather your personal best measurement so that you can use this as a benchmark for comparing your measurements in the future. How do you identify your personal best or baseline? By taking multiple readings while you are well and problem free. I guide my patients to do so by taking peak flow readings two times a day for a week. The highest value represents their personal best.

Once you know your personal best peak flow reading, you will be able to interpret future results when you use the meter. Although you can get an idea of where your normal value should be from a standardized table or formulas, it seems to be better to establish your peak flow baseline in a more individualized way. The personal best number is yours alone. It fits you perfectly.

MAKING SENSE OF PEAK FLOW READINGS

How do you interpret a peak flow reading?

If your peak flow is within 80% or greater than your personal best, you are said to be in your green zone. If you are feeling well, no additional action steps are needed.

If your peak flow is 20-50% less than your personal best, this suggests a problem is there or coming. You have to begin treatment and perhaps seek medical advice.

If your peak flow is less than 50% of your personal best peak flow measurement, you need to seek immediate attention, especially if you are having symptoms such as cough, wheezing, or chest tightness. (This ties into your asthma action plan, which we will review in Chapter 8.)

It is important not to get too fixated on the peak-flow-meter number alone; if everything is fine, and you are having no symptoms, and the peak flow is a bit low, it's probably not your asthma acting up. Because peak flow is effort-dependent, this happens in adults and children who are sick and tired without the energy needed to perform a good measurement. Having said that, it is important to be absolutely certain that this low number is not part of a serious asthma attack.

In the past, it has been suggested that everyone with asthma perform regular peak flow measurements. The pendulum in asthma care now seems to be swinging away from that recommendation and toward a more targeted use of peak flow measurements.

So, how is the peak flow meter most helpful?

It is especially good for those who have trouble recognizing when asthma problems are developing; in these cases, it may be reasonable to take peak flow measurements every day.

In my experience, most people with asthma are in touch with their body signals. That is, they recognize early warning signs of worsening asthma such as chest tightness, cough, and subtle wheezing, and they act on them quickly. This feeling of difficulty breathing is known as dyspnea (disp-nea). While most people are capable of perceiving this feeling as it develops, there are others, at both ends of the spectrum, who cannot. These individuals can be classified into those people with:

- low perception of dyspnea (POD)
- high POD.

PEOPLE WITH LOW POD

Individuals with low POD don't recognize that their lung function is falling. They typically say they are feeling fine, but when you measure lung function, their values are reduced by 20–30% of normal. They are not fine, but they don't recognize it. As a result, they are at risk of developing much more severe symptoms and asthma attacks that seem to come out of nowhere. Using regular peak flow measurements can be useful here because as the numbers fall, it will give them an early warning of developing problems. It will help them learn to connect what they feel with low lung function. The idea is to help them recognize problems and begin treatment earlier.

PEOPLE WITH HIGH POD

On the other end of the spectrum, you have people with a high POD who are oversensitive to very small changes in their lungs. They tend to overuse their bronchodilator inhaler. I most often see this in adolescents who are overreaching for their inhaler, using it without clearly needing to. Perhaps this is because these active young people are machines in motion who are prone to react with the best quick fix they know. Regardless of the reason for high POD, it's preferable to have a more accurate understanding of how to read one's body signals. The peak flow meter can provide that.

For example, if someone with high POD uses the peak flow meter, he or she may learn to tune into asthma symptoms better and use short-acting medicines only when necessary. The benefit of avoiding overuse of these short-acting medicines is that a person's body will then remain sensitive to the bronchodilator inhaler when they need it and avoid side effects such as jitteriness or irritability.

So, if you fall into one of these two categories (high or low POD), regularly using a peak flow meter may be just what the doctor orders!

PULSE OXIMETER

This is a handy little tool that easily and non-invasively measures the level of oxygen in your blood—no pins, no needles, no injections. The level of oxygen in your blood is one of the first things you will see falling as an asthma attack develops. So, if you suspect asthma is worsening, the pulse oximeter can help confirm that for you.

At my practice, we measure pulse oximetry at every office visit for all of our asthmatic patients, much as a family physician might take a blood pressure readings. The pulse oximeter is also used in Emergency Rooms and for hospitalized patients with asthma to get a quick sense of what's going on.

One child's parents bought a pulse oximeter for home use several years ago. I don't routinely recommend doing this, but in this child the parents really had a difficult time recognizing early the onset of acute asthma problems. Dad noted that his daughter had not required an emergency visit since they began using it! In this situation, the pulse oximeter really helped the parents recognize problems and begin treatment earlier.

When the pulse oximeter reading comes back normal, it is highly reassuring to both patient and doctor that all is well. When the reading comes back below normal, it is a cue that further exploration should be done.

Now, the information that the pulse oximeter provides is helpful, but most of the time it just confirms what we already know, especially when we are certain we are dealing with an acute asthma attack. In addition, the number by itself is not a cause for panic. It is just one piece of information that tells you how someone is doing.

I have seen healthcare workers become so entranced by this number that they forget to look at the whole picture. They may forget that there is a person attached to this number, that the reading should be taken in the context of the whole person. Your doctor should ask, are you having difficulty breathing? How badly? Are you able to carry on a conversation easily? Are you getting better or worse? I am not against this technologic advance as long as we healthcare practitioners don't forget the obvious. Make sure your doctor looks at the entire picture! Make sure your doctor looks at the whole person and the disease process!

EXHALED NITRIC OXIDE (ENO)

One of the newer tests is the eNO test. This test measures the amount of nitric oxide present in the air that is exhaled.

Why is this reading of interest? Because nitric oxide (a gas) is produced in the lungs when inflammation is present. It can be easily measured. The greater the inflammation present, the higher the amount of NO exhaled. Recalling that inflammation is one of the major problems in the lungs of someone with asthma, you can see how this measurement might be a useful monitoring tool. As asthma worsens eNO rises.

The eNO test is not in widespread use at the present time. Well-respected asthma researchers have reported that using these measurements may add no more value over closely following the NIH-sponsored asthma treatment guidelines.[1] If the cost of conducting the eNO test were to decline, its use might increase. For now, there has not been widespread adoption of this particular tool. Recent asthma guidelines published by the American Thoracic Society have recommended the routine use of measuring eNO in monitoring asthma, so we may see its use grow.

To sum it up, there are measurements of pulmonary function that are helpful in the management of asthma. The use of PFTs is considered standard of care for asthma, and any comprehensive asthma care plan needs to include them in its toolbox. Measurement of peak flow can be helpful, too, especially in those who are over- or under-sensitive to the symptoms that signal worsening asthma. These tools are one part of the plan in helping you to beat asthma. Stay on top of your current lung function with these tests, and you and your doctor will have the information you need to give you standout treatment.

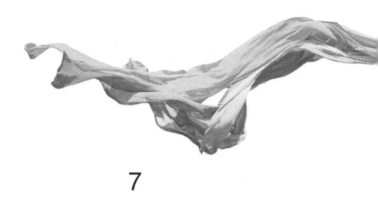

7

Pharmaceuticals

Thinking about the treatment of asthma, I oftentimes look upon it as a piece of music. Does this sound silly? Well, for me, asthma treatment is a little bit like a symphony. Once you get the gist of what I mean here, your imagination may see it the same way, or perhaps you will see it as other music. Rock. Blues. Bluegrass. Rap. Opera. Hip-hop. Whatever your taste in music, try to imagine this with me.

All music has an underlying beat or rhythm. In asthma treatment, I see this underlying "beat" as being the basic treatment plan used daily to treat asthma. This day-in, day-out maintenance of asthma control is like the beat–beat–beat rhythm in a piece of music.

At different times in a musical piece, the music becomes louder or softer, harsh or mellow, heavenly or dark. Different instruments or voices are brought in and out to make the perfect whole. The rhythm changes. This is much like asthma symptoms themselves, which will vary over time in response to the different triggers you face. In response, different types and amounts of medicine will need to be started or stopped.

The treatment of asthma is like a musical balancing act, in which there is a balance of drums, horns, guitar, etc. In asthma, that balance happens through the use of different medications—just enough of each...not too little, not too much. In the end, it is an integrated whole. Each piece makes sense; each piece has its proper place.

For example, I recently saw a patient who has severe asthma. In addition to multiple medications, we had started a fairly new biologic drug called omalizumab (Xolair), which is given by injection every 2–4 weeks. He was improving on this new medication. However, since our last office visit months earlier, feeling well, he had stopped all of his other asthma drugs and again began to experience progressively worsening symptoms. Clearly, his approach of stopping his other asthma medications was unsuccessful.

This example illustrates several issues. First, it demonstrates the importance of the stepped approach to asthma therapy, which we will cover in this chapter. Second, it shows the need for a collaborative relationship between patient and physician, which we will cover in Chapter 9. Third, it shows the need for persistence and consistency. Suffice it to say for now that, when dealing with a complicated disease like asthma, decisions are made best by the patient and physician together, not independently.

In this chapter, we will cover the concepts of understanding the severity of your asthma, asthma control and how these relate to the medicines you may be prescribed. Then, we will look at the approach to treating asthma with medications using what is known as "step therapy." Finally, we will do a brief review of the various pharmaceutical agents commonly used in treating asthma today so you have the knowledge you need to recognize and understand the medications your doctor is (or is not) prescribing for you. The ultimate goal is to get the musical balancing act of asthma treatment—whether it involves one, two, three medications, or more—flowing in perfect harmony.

UNDERSTANDING ASTHMA
SEVERITY AND CONTROL

When you first begin seeing a doctor for your asthma, he or she will want to assess the severity of your asthma: how often does your asthma cause problems and how serious are these problems? The doctor will begin by assessing whether your asthma is intermittent or persistent.

People with intermittent asthma have asthma symptoms twice a week or less, use a bronchodilator inhaler twice a week or less (not counting treating exercise-associated asthma symptoms), have no interference with their daily activities, and have no nighttime asthma symptoms.

In contrast, people with persistent asthma have symptoms more than two days a week as well as at night, use their bronchodilator inhaler more than two days a week, experience interference with daily activities, and have two or more asthma attacks in a year that require the use of oral steroids.

If your asthma is intermittent, it will not take too much medicine to control it. If your asthma is persistent, you should expect your doctor will work up a more complex plan for your medication regimen (the details of which we will see in the stepped therapy approach described later in this chapter).

In my opinion, far too many individuals are erroneously diagnosed as having intermittent asthma and are undertreated as a result. This inaccurate diagnosis—and thus lack of appropriate pharmaceutical treatment—causes many more individuals with asthma to suffer than should be the case. Once someone is empowered to understand the true state of his or her asthma (e.g., persistent vs. intermittent, controlled vs. uncontrolled), he or she will have the information needed to seek the appropriate level of treatment.

What are the practical applications of knowing one's asthma severity when it comes to deciding which asthma medicines will be used? Individuals with intermittent asthma will generally only require a bronchodilator inhaler such as albuterol or levalbuterol. Those with persistent asthma will be treated with the same initial medication plus increasing strengths and numbers of medications as needed.

As it turns out, your asthma severity is only one piece of the puzzle when it comes to determining the correct asthma medicines for you to use. As noted in the Asthma Guidelines Expert Panel report,

> Once therapy is initiated, the emphasis thereafter for clinical management is changed to the assessment of *asthma control* [emphasis added]. The level of asthma control will guide decisions either to maintain or adjust therapy.

In other words, once you start treatment, your physician will move from a focus on asthma severity to asthma control. This is just another way of understanding and analyzing your asthma, and it is a very practical one due to its simplicity: Your asthma is either under control or not.

You are either moving easily through your life, much like your friends who don't have asthma (controlled asthma), or you are suffering uncomfortable, maybe even frightening, asthma symptoms that reduce your quality of life (uncontrolled asthma).

How does this information about controlled versus uncontrolled asthma help your doctor create your medication plan? When your asthma moves to uncontrolled, you and your doctor will step up your medications (e.g., increase dosage, add more medications). When your asthma comes back under control, you and your doctor will step you down off some medications. The most important information for you to take from here is that the state of your asthma control will determine the approach to medication therapy.

After asthma is diagnosed and initial treatment begins, the focus then shifts to the following question: Is your asthma in control or out of control?

If your asthma is controlled, no further action is necessary (other than considering whether the amount of therapy can be reduced or not). Stay the course. Continue doing what you are doing. If your asthma is uncontrolled, then evaluation and action are needed. Therapy may need to be changed.

GETTING STARTED ON
ASSESSING MEDICATIONS

When you first see the doctor for help with your asthma, you may be anxious to get on new or different medications right away. But before increasing or adding new medications, evaluation should always come first. Important questions your doctor should ask include:

- Are you being exposed to a new irritant or allergen?
- Do you have a sinusitis or other infection?
- Are you having problems with reflux or "GERD" (heartburn)?

- Are you correctly taking your current medications as prescribed (adherence)?

These issues should be dealt with first, before any changes to long-term medication therapy are made.

Don't Forget to Take Your Medicine!

This may seem silly, but the question of adherence must be considered when asthma is difficult to control. Physicians commonly assume that most patients adhere to their medication regimen as prescribed. The truth is that this is often not the case. Many people do not stick to the plan after they start to feel better.

Knowing what you know now, you understand the need to take your medications as prescribed! If you have difficulties with this, they should be honestly discussed with your physician. Whether it is financial issues or problems with medication taste or side effects, you may be able to brainstorm an answer together. It is far better to correctly and maximally use one medication before adding an additional medication with its inherent risks and side effects.

"Why did this attack happen now?" is a question that always needs to be answered when you become ill. If you understand why it happened, you have gained valuable insight that may help you to prevent a future problem.

Now, let's look at how you and your doctor can approach asthma control in terms of adding and reducing medications.

STEP THERAPY

Step therapy is a basic approach to using medications in treating asthma. You step up (add additional medications) to achieve control over asthma. Once control is achieved, you maintain that number of medications for 6–12 months. This gives the lungs the needed time to recover from inflammation. Then, you step down therapy (reducing the number or strength of medications used) over a period of time, watching to be sure that you maintain control. You then stay on that lowest step or level of medications (again, my approach is at least 6 months) before attempting to step down any further.

If at any time during the period of stepping down, asthma begins to worsen, you will step up the level of therapy to regain control, before attempting to step down any further. This is fine-tuning asthma control, and it requires patience.

For example, you start asthma treatment with a basic short-acting bronchodilator inhaler (albuterol, for example). If the asthma is controlled, you hold at that level of medication. If asthma is still not controlled you step up to the next level of medication, adding an inhaled steroid inhaler such as momentasone (Asmanex) or a pill called montelukast (Singulair). If symptoms are controlled, you hold at that level of medication. In a minority of asthma cases, the disease is so severe that you need multiple medications (all the way up to daily oral steroids) before control is achieved.

The good news?

Most patients with asthma are able to achieve control with one or two maintenance (daily) medications. Most people do not have severe disease and therefore require far fewer medications than people with much worse asthma.

YOUR GUIDE TO ASTHMA MEDICATIONS

You may recall the analogy used at the beginning of this chapter—that asthma treatment is like a symphony. Just as the music may grow louder or softer, so too may your doctor intensify your asthma treatment by adding medicines or pulling back when ready by removing medicines from your regimen. That is what we just saw in the case of step therapy. Similarly, as there are different musical instruments (string, percussion, woodwind, and so on) played in a symphony to create varying desired effects, there are also different medications available to you and your doctor for treating your asthma.

The medicines available for asthma treatment can be categorized into two groups: those used to help you when you are having acute symptoms, like cough, wheezing, and chest tightness, and those taken daily to keep the illness controlled. The first group of medicines, for acute situations, are sometimes called reliever or rescue medications, though I like the term "bronchodilator medications" for this category.

The second group of medicines are referred to as "controller medications." I prefer the term "maintenance medications" because they should be used every day!

Bronchodilator medications. Bronchodilator medications are intended for use when an asthma attack occurs, when asthma symptoms worsen, or to prevent exercise-induced asthma. When asthma is well controlled, bronchodilator medications should be needed twice a week or less. They are the basic component of your toolkit and are the only medications needed by the small number of people with the mildest form of asthma (intermittent) or those with purely exercise-induced asthma. Bronchodilator medications can be administered by the patient (or parents) when needed.

How do bronchodilator medications work? They cause the smooth muscle of the airways to relax, thereby reducing the cough, wheezing, and chest tightness that may be felt with an asthma attack. (Think back to Chapter 3, "Understanding the Problem.") They do this by binding to a receptor on the smooth muscle of the airways (called a beta receptor). In medical jargon, they are known as beta agonists. They are found as short-acting (lasting 4-6 hours) or long-acting (working for up to 12 hours). The short-acting bronchodilators are used for acute asthma symptoms or to prevent exercise-induced symptoms. The long-acting bronchodilators are used in asthma only in combination inhalers, which include an inhaled corticosteroid medication also.

Bronchodilator medications are delivered either by an inhaler or a nebulizer. Using the correct technique with them is, of course, important. See the appendix for instructions on correct use of inhalers.

The most common side effect of bronchodilator medications is jitteriness, which can be quite uncomfortable for some people. This happens because these medications stimulate the skeletal muscles in the arms and legs as well as the muscles in the lungs. They may also cause the heart rate to increase by stimulating the heart muscle.

Albuterol is the generic name for the bronchodilator medication most commonly used. Common brand names include Proventil, Ventolin, and ProAir; a newer variant is called levalbuterol (Xopenex), which may produce less uncomfortable side effects. No generic form of bronchodilator medicine was available at the writing of this book.

If the asthma episode becomes particularly extreme and the patient ends up in the doctor's office or the hospital, a drug known as ipratropium (Atrovent) may be used (an anti-cholinergic drug).

Anti-inflammatory medications. Drugs in this class of medication include inhaled steroids, oral pills, inhalers that combine steroids with long-acting bronchodilators (combination inhalers), and medications given by injection.

Inhaled steroids. Inhaled steroid medications block a number of different mediators or biochemical reactions in the lungs. What does that mean in regular terms? It means that inhaled steroids reduce inflammation and twitchiness in the airways. Inhaled steroids are anti-inflammatory medications.

From an earlier chapter on the problems found in the asthmatic lungs, you may recall that inflammation plays a key role in asthma. Inhaled steroids are probably the most commonly used medications in treating the inflammation that comes with persistent asthma. They are usually the medications next added for those with persistent disease or when asthma can't be controlled by using bronchodilator medications alone.

Once begun, these medications must be used *daily*. Unlike albuterol, they are not intended to be used on an as-needed basis. In fact, they may take a month of steady use to be completely effective. That being said, I prefer to use them over 6–12 months with good asthma control before stepping down off of them. It has been shown that it may take this long for all of the inflammation in the lungs to be completely cleared.

Inhaled steroids are delivered through a metered-dose inhaler, dry powdered inhaler, or nebulizer.

Common side effects include mouth and tongue irritation, vocal cord irritation, and hoarseness. It's important to maintain good oral hygiene when using these drugs. Simply rinsing the mouth out after taking the medication usually suffices. If hoarseness occurs as a side effect, it may need to be addressed by switching to a different medication or, when possible, reducing the dose. Also, the use of a small chamber called a spacer, which fits onto the end of the inhaler, may be used to help reduce these symptoms as well.

There are a number of different medication choices available for delivery through inhalers, including momentasone (Asmanex), fluticasone (Flovent), beclomethasone (Q-var), and budesonide (Pulmicort). Budesonide is also available in a form that can be delivered by a nebulizer.

To Use Steroids or Not to Use Steroids

There is sometimes a desire, especially on the part of parents, to not want to use inhaled steroids because of fear of the potential side effects such as interference with normal growth, hypertension, and cataracts among others. Of course, no medication is devoid of potential side effects. Yet, the risk to the patient or child who needs inhaled steroids and does not take them can be far greater than the risks of the inhaled steroids themselves.

Inhaled steroids are different from *oral steroids*. Inhaled steroids tend to work at the surface of the lung with less absorption into the body. They primarily work right where they are needed. In contrast, oral steroids must travel through the entire body to reach the lungs.

text block continues...

To Use Steroids or Not to Use Steroids continued...

In addition, because they are used in higher doses, oral steroids tend to be more prone to causing side effects. Inhaled steroids are much safer than oral steroids.

I want parents especially to consider what they are choosing when they decide not to use inhaled steroids in treating asthma. This often equates to choosing to have uncontrolled asthma, with nighttime episodes, trips to the ER, and severe asthma attacks, as well as long-term potential damage to lung growth and structure. We must be aware of the law of unintended consequences.

By choosing to use inhaled steroids when prescribed, you are more likely to avoid the need to use oral steroids down the road when asthma worsens. That's important information to consider!

Anti-inflammatory pills. Unlike the inhaled steroid medications, which block a number of different mediator reactions in the lungs—that is, reduce inflammation and twitchiness in the airways—what I refer to as anti-inflammatory pills target a narrow area involved in airway twitchiness only. It's like the difference between the beam from a searchlight (the inhaled steroids) and a laser beam, which is more narrowly targeted (anti-inflammatory pills).

The two most common drugs in this class in use today include montelukast (Singulair) and zileuton (Zyflo CR).

Montelukast may be used in children or adults. Zileuton is used for adults and children over 12.

Montelukast is the more commonly prescribed of the two. It comes in a granulated form (for younger children) and in a tablet form that can be chewed or swallowed. It may be used as a second step in treating asthma. It is my perception that parents of children with asthma may be more inclined to try this medication first because of their concerns over the use of inhaled steroids. In fact, I have treated many patients (children especially) who have been helped by this medication. It does not seem to be effective in everyone, though, for reasons that are not clear. I see few problems in giving it a trial for a month, as long as it is discontinued if it isn't effective in that time frame.

Montelukast (Singulair) is considered to be a fairly safe medication. In some patients, though, it has been associated with psychiatric problems (depression, mood changes) and should be stopped if these problems appear. If you (or your child) experience such problems, you should consult your physician immediately.

A doctor may add zileuton to a patient's medications if the patient hasn't yet achieved asthma control—that is, for people who are using a bronchodilator inhaler, inhaled steroid medicines, *and/or* combination inhalers (more on these in the next section) but still need additional treatment. If zileuton is used, liver function must be periodically monitored with blood tests since it may cause liver inflammation.

Combination inhalers. These medications combine an inhaled steroid and a long-acting bronchodilator (also known as LABA) into one inhaler. The LABA acts much like the short-acting bronchodilator medications we covered previously; however, the effects of these long-acting drugs last for 12 rather than 4–6 hours! There are three such medications available at the time of this writing: Advair, which combines fluticasone (Flovent) with salmeterol (Serevent); Symbicort, combining budesonide (Pulmicort) and formoterol (Foradil); and Dulera, containing momentasone (Asmanex) and formoterol.

When asthma is not controlled using inhaled steroid medications, combination inhalers are usually the next step up in therapy. There are three important things to remember about these medications:

1. They are to be added only when inhaled steroids are not completely effective.

2. They are not approved in the United States for use as a bronchodilator in treating acute asthma problems.

3. The U.S. Food and Drug Administration (FDA) has required a boxed-warning label on these medications stating that their use may result in *death*.

Point number 3 is bound to get your attention. It gets mine. This is known as a class warning. It applies to all medications containing LABAs. It is a warning I believe we should take seriously. It reminds us that there is no absolutely risk-free medication. Physicians should not use these drugs in a cavalier manner. They should be used when needed and stepped down from when they clearly are no longer necessary.

But, let's not throw the baby out with the bathwater! I believe the risks are very low if this drug is used correctly (in combination with an inhaled steroid). In fact, there is strong belief in our medical community that the initial study reporting deaths from LABA had some significant issues in the way it was conducted.[1] Since these drugs were first introduced, the number of annual deaths from asthma in the United States has fallen, if anything. To my mind, I would expect the number of deaths to have risen if these were truly "toxic" drugs. So, I believe we should continue to use them *when needed* to gain effective control over asthma.

Possible side effects include, among others, those mentioned for inhaled steroids, plus jitteriness due to the LABA component.

Combination inhalers come in varying strengths, with the patient taking the medication via aerosol (metered-dose inhaler) or a dry powder that is inhaled (breath-actuated dry-powder inhaler). Patients may do better with the metered-dose inhalers if the dry powdered type is too irritating.

What is next if these medications are not effective? At this point, we are at the level of asthma that is considered persistent and severe. This level of asthma is relatively rare and extremely difficult to control, with fewer and fewer treatment options. Unfortunately, even with maximum therapy, individuals in this group may experience symptoms every day.

People with this severe level of asthma may require oral steroids, such as prednisone. Through daily or every-other-day dosing, individuals in this group may be able to achieve control of their asthma. Although oral steroids may be effective, and are commonly used to treat acute exacerbations, they are not without significant side effects: cataract development, personality changes, bone loss, high blood pressure, diabetes, and stretch marks on the skin. Our ultimate aim is to reduce the need for oral steroids when we can. There is hope for these most severe patients in the use of the medications listed below—as well as other medications that are in development.

Omalizumab (Xolair). This drug is currently approved for patients with more severe allergic asthma. Xolair works by binding with and removing allergy antibodies, thus reducing allergic reactions. At the present time, this drug is not approved for patients with non-allergic asthma.

Typically, Xolair is given by an injection once or twice a month. In part because this drug is costly (at the time this book was written, the drug cost up to thousands of dollars a month to administer), patients have to meet certain requirements to be eligible for using this medicine, including poorly controlled asthma, an elevated total blood allergy antibody level within a defined range, and certain body weight limits.

When those criteria are in place, Xolair is typically effective. Its major drawbacks include the need to administer it under medical supervision by injection and its cost. The manufacturer and other pharmaceutical companies have developed financial aid programs for patients who need it but can't afford it. Although current guidelines make it clear as to when it is appropriate to consider using Xolair, it is not clear as to when, if ever, the drug can be stopped. More work needs to be done to better understand the drug's use.

Again, as with all pharmaceuticals, side effects may occur when taking Xolair. For example, evaluation of earlier studies with this drug link it with an increased risk of cancer. Researchers still cannot explain this finding away, nor should doctors and patients sweep it under the rug. Researchers are monitoring patients treated with this medication to evaluate the real risk. There also appears to be an increased risk of a severe allergic reaction after the administration of this medication (anaphylaxis). Clearly, the risks, costs, and potential benefits with this drug must be carefully weighed on a case-by-case basis. In the near future, we will probably see additional newer biopharmaceutical agents approved for use in the struggle against asthma.

IMMUNOTHERAPY

I would be remiss as an allergist if I did not mention the use of immunotherapy in asthma. Immunotherapy, commonly known as allergy shots or IT, is a tool in the allergist's toolbox that can be very helpful in treating nasal allergies and asthma. Allergy to pollens, animal dander, and so on can cause nasal symptoms such as itchy nose, sneezing, and nasal congestion. By causing nasal problems, allergens can indirectly make asthma worse, but also may produce asthma symptoms by directly stimulating an allergic reaction in the lungs.

The use of high-dose immunotherapy is well documented in the medical literature as an effective treatment of both nasal allergic disease and allergic asthma and is considered safe.[2] It appears to work by a complex mechanism that includes restoring a certain balance of cells and mediators in the body away from the imbalance that is associated with allergic disease.

The current standard of care for allergy shots involves injections, once or twice a week for a couple of months, then once weekly, then less often as time progresses. It can also be administered by a clustered dosing schedule or "RUSH" therapy, both designed to progress more rapidly to the maintenance doses. A complete course of IT lasts for 3-5 years.

Currently, research is underway on administering IT orally. It is not yet approved for general use in the United

States, although some of my allergist colleagues are attempting to use it in some of their patients' care by mixing the extracts we already have available to us into oral serums delivered in drop form. Oral IT is more commonly used in Europe.

Would I like to get rid of all the needles in my office? Absolutely. But for now, I am waiting to see scientific data on the safety and effectiveness of oral IT, as well as the presence of standardized oral IT products in the U.S. marketplace before using or recommending it to my patients.

The most common side effect of allergy shots is local reactions, such as local redness or swelling, but severe allergic reactions (anaphylaxis) and death can also occur—although these are rare. Having active asthma symptoms at the time of injection appears to be a significant risk factor for a fatal reaction after allergy shots.

It is thus extremely important to remember that, if you have asthma and are on immunotherapy, never take an injection if your asthma is currently or recently causing you problems (i.e., coughing, wheezing, chest tightness etc.)

To not follow this rule increases your risk of death after an allergy injection. Thus, it is important to get your asthma taken care of first and then resume your injections only as and when your physician recommends.

Allergy shots should only be administered under direct medical supervision in a facility equipped to handle anaphylaxis. This is the currently accepted standard of care. It is inconvenient, but if you have an allergic reaction, expert and immediate medical care is the best way to stop it.

One of the most exciting developments in understanding the use of allergy shots is the possibility that they may play a role in *preventing* asthma in children. As stated in the Guidelines for the use of IT:

> Immunotherapy for children is effective and often well tolerated. Therefore immunotherapy should be considered (along with pharmacotherapy and allergen avoidance) in the management of children with allergic rhinitis, allergic asthma, and stinging insect hypersensitivity. It might prevent the new onset of allergen sensitivities or *progression to asthma*.[3] (emphasis added)

Research has demonstrated that treatment of allergies with allergy shots—in addition to standard measures such as avoidance and medications—significantly reduced the later development of asthma in those children who used IT over children treated using standard measures alone. To me, this is real food for thought when faced with children experiencing bad allergy symptoms who are at increased risk of developing asthma (such as having a parent with a history of asthma).

Well, dear reader, we have covered quite a bit of information in this chapter. Hopefully, you can now better understand how asthma is classified, whether it is controlled or not, and how various medications are utilized in treating this complex disease. On to the Asthma Action plan!

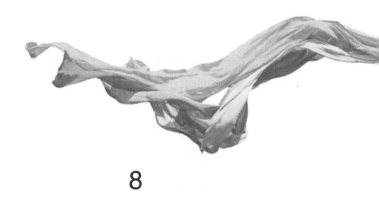

8

The Asthma Action Plan

Tom Landry, the legendary coach of the Dallas Cowboys, once said, "Setting a goal is not the main thing. It is deciding how you will go about achieving it and staying with that plan." I completely agree, and, putting it into my own words: You just gotta have a plan! (Just so we agree, Coach Landry said it better, but I used fewer words!)

The simple truth is, when your asthma is under control, the plan is easy: Keep doing what you're doing. I like that approach and I suspect you do as well. However, as you know all too well, the good times never seem to last as long as we would like them to. Triggers come and triggers go, leaving uncontrolled asthma in their wake. You must have a plan of action for what to do when those difficult times come, and the best plans are laid out well in advance.

Let me illuminate this point with something I learned some years ago, while I was a physician in the United States Air Force. Some of my time during that period was spent as a flight surgeon, which involved working with fighter pilots, remarkable people to be certain. Fighter pilots spend a considerable amount of time training to do their job. In fact, they train for every possible contingency, over and over again. As a result, their actions and reactions become hard-wired reflexes.

One critical decision—when to eject from a fighter jet in a time of emergency—is best made long before the pilots have to do it. In their situation of hurtling along at supersonic speed, the pilots may have seconds or even a fraction of a second in which to make a correct decision. This can be a matter of life or death for them. This is why this decision must be made well in advance.

When facing this decision, fighter pilots don't hesitate; they do what they planned long before: When the conditions indicate it's necessary, they pull the eject lever and punch out. (As I heard one of them once wryly remark, "This is called giving the plane back to the taxpayer," tongue in cheek, of course!). Quick action saves these pilots' lives, even if, unfortunately, the jet is lost.

Thankfully, most of the decisions we have to make with asthma do not have to be made within a few seconds, as with those of a fighter pilot. Nonetheless, the decisions you have to make when your asthma starts to tilt out of control are extremely important and need to be made correctly and in a timely fashion. Just as with a fighter pilot, these decisions should be made ahead of time. This is where the asthma action plan comes into play.

YOUR ROADMAP: THE ASTHMA ACTION PLAN

What is an asthma action plan? Think of it as a roadmap or a guide, with everything in one place that you will need for a trip. Controlled asthma is your destination, and the asthma action plan will get you there. This plan is intended to promote early intervention when things go wrong.

The asthma action plan can be simple or complex, written or unwritten, very detailed or short and straightforward. It all depends on what works best for you. Having the plan written down can be especially helpful to those of us who are somewhat disorganized or who can't seem to recall the plan information quickly from memory. The important point is to have a plan and "stay with it," to paraphrase Coach Landry.

SIGNALS AND YOUR ACTION PLAN

Perhaps the most common asthma action plan in use today is based on three zones that are given traffic-signal colors:

green, yellow, and red. These zones are correlated with signs or symptoms of asthma as well as with action steps that should be taken. Let's look at how this all works.

In the green zone, you see that:

- your breathing is good
- you have no cough or wheeze
- you are able to sleep through the night
- you are able to work and play normally.

No action step, other than using all of your medications as prescribed, is necessary.

In medical terms, the green zone corresponds with a peak flow reading of 80% or greater of your personal best. Back in Chapter 6 we saw that peak flow is a measurement of your lung function, using a small medical device, the peak flow meter. The better the lungs are functioning, the higher the peak flow level. You will know you are in the green zone either by taking your peak flow reading or by observing the lack of asthma symptoms, as described above.

After the green zone comes the yellow zone. The yellow zone is extremely important, in my mind. The decisions you make here will affect how bad things get and how quickly you recover. Much like the fighter pilot, you must be ready and respond.

If your asthma is in the yellow zone, you may find that you have:

- the first signs of a cold or allergies
- coughing
- mild wheezing
- tightness in your chest
- coughing at night.

When you are in the yellow zone, it is also possible that you've had recent exposure to a known asthma trigger.

In the yellow zone, your peak flow level will fall within 50–80% of your personal best. It is here that your asthma is clearly beginning to worsen. In other words, you are having an asthma attack (asthma flare-up or exacerbation). Action is necessary and should be taken right now—not later—because time is of the essence here. The longer problems go untreated in the yellow zone, the harder they become to fix.

Typically, your asthma action plan in the yellow zone would involve:

- removing yourself from the presence of the allergic asthma trigger
- taking two puffs of your short-acting bronchodilator or using your asthma nebulizer.

Many times, your symptoms will reverse in response to such action and your peak flow will return to your green zone. Your bronchodilator inhaler and removal of asthma trigger will have been all that was necessary.

But, if symptoms persist, taking a second dose of your bronchodilator inhaler or nebulizer makes sense, and then using it as needed up to 4 times daily for a few days, but only if the attack is not worsening. Many physicians, myself included, would also like you to call us at that time, even if things stabilize. Further steps, such as an office visit, medication adjustment, or inclusion of additional medications (i.e., steroids, antibiotics) may be needed. Sometimes a course of oral steroids may be kept at home to begin if needed over a weekend or holiday to get a head start on treatment.

The idea is not to try and go it alone here, especially if the diagnosis of asthma is fairly new to you. Both you and your physician are learning about how your asthma behaves, and an office visit helps facilitate that learning process.

Calling or visiting your doctor at this point also ensures that you can together make the necessary adjustments to your *long-term* treatment plan, helping you go beyond the acute treatment that was given to stabilize you when you entered the yellow zone. That is, together you can try to determine why you fell into the yellow zone. This negative progression from green to yellow may be a sign that your overall treatment plan needs adjusting.

Now, what if you find yourself in the red zone? In this case, your peak flow is less than 50% of your personal best and your asthma is quickly getting worse. You may find that:

- your bronchodilator medicine is not helping you to feel any better
- your breathing is hard and fast
- your nose opens wide as you breathe
- as you breathe in, your ribs show
- you are unable to talk easily
- your lips, skin, or fingernails become dusky or blue.

What do you do if you find yourself in the red zone?

Using the example of the fighter pilot, the time has come to pull the lever and eject. This is an absolute emergency, and there is no time to waste. Your emergency lever is the telephone, and 911 are the numbers you call to punch out. Yes, in the red zone, you must call 911 and you must do it now. This is no time to worry about calling attention to yourself and it is no time to go it alone. It is also not the time for those around you to sit and calmly analyze the situation. This is a time for action.

I want you to plan for this possibility now, long before it ever happens. You most likely will be confused and frightened if it occurs, and you may not be thinking clearly. You must decide now that, if you ever find yourself in the bad situation I described above, you will call 911 or have someone call for you!

Take some time now to review those symptoms so you are able to recognize when you are in the red zone. You might even want to post the symptoms somewhere where it's easy to review them from time to time, like the inside door of a commonly used kitchen cabinet or the front of your weekly planner. If you have a written asthma action plan, the symptoms of the red zone can be written there.

Having said all that, I want to reinforce that we want to do everything in our power to prevent you from entering the dreaded red zone. This is why taking your daily medications as prescribed is so important. This is why your actions in the yellow zone are so important. This is why having a plan is so important.

Thus, your green–yellow–red zone asthma plan looks at a combination of your peak flow levels plus the presence of asthma symptoms and distress to identify your current asthma state; it then couples those items with specific action steps for you to take. I have provided a link to this type of plan as recommended by the Allergy & Asthma Foundation of America in the footnote below.* You can also go to the *Beating Asthma* book website (www.beatingasthma.com) to download an asthma action plan to review with your physician. We are also working to develop a simple asthma action-plan iPhone app that allows you to carry this useful tool with you wherever you go.

_____

* http://aafa.org/pdfs/AsthmaActionPlan.pdf

REAL-WORLD APPROACH
TO ASTHMA ACTION PLANS

Given that I have mentioned that your asthma action plan can be written or verbal, you might be wondering how I help my patients select the right choice for them. Fair question.

All of my patients have an asthma action plan. Some are written; some are not. I believe in using simple straightforward advice. I explain to all my asthma patients this plan. "If you break the Rules of Two, call me. If you are having asthma symptoms that don't go away by using bronchodilator medication, call me."

Now, if someone is consistently coming in sick and I can see that they are not calling me early, I say, "Let's get it written down," and I give them a written action plan. If the person has problems sensing when his or her asthma is worsening, they get a peak flow meter also.

Two final points to consider.

First, many people find that they experience some unique sensation or symptom that tells them very early that their asthma is about to flare. Some people experience an itching of skin on the front of their neck before their asthma acts up. Some parents notice their children become unusually quiet before their asthma flares. I encourage you to be sensitive to and watch for these indicators in yourself. If you experience something like these early warning signs, use them to your advantage and begin following your asthma action plan.

Second, if you have to make an acute visit to an Emergency Room or Acute Care type office for an asthma attack, let your allergist or personal physician know about that visit within two days. This will allow you to head off problems that need further attention. Why? It allows you to close the loop with the physician who knows you best, making certain that going forward, your treatment plan is correctly suited to your needs.

I hope I have conveyed to you the key role that an asthma action plan plays in helping you to beat asthma. Without an understanding of what you will do when your asthma flares up, you are at the mercy of asthma. Having an asthma action plan empowers you.

Let's move along to discuss the topic of your relationship with your physician.

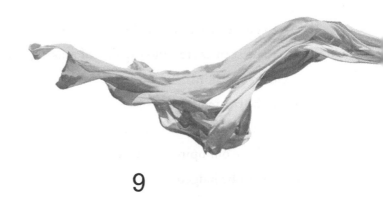

9

The Patient–Physician Relationship

If I were to ask you what your expectations were for the relationships in your life, what would you say? How do you think others should interact with you, how should they treat you, and how should they view you? I imagine that, if we were to ask this question of 100 or 1,000 or 1 million people, we would get many unique answers. I suspect, however, that there would be many common expectations that most of us, as human beings, would agree upon. I think we all expect to be treated with common human decency from others. For example, we all want:

- to be treated as human beings, not objects
- to be seen as free and capable of making our own decisions
- to be treated fairly
- to be treated with respect
- to have our opinions heard
- to not be judged.

Some of us might add some things to this list, perhaps some things unique to each of us as individuals. For the sake of discussion, though, let's say that these are the common things we all expect from each other. If we adhere to the Golden Rule—to do to others as we want them to do to us—then we realize that if we expect these things from others, we have to treat them in this way as well.

Do we always meet this standard? Heck no! At least, I know that I don't. As human beings, we may strive for perfection but rarely if ever do we reach it. Being human means that we are imperfect; we have our weaknesses, our faults, and our fears. Our human frailties can get in the way of our positive interaction with others. We don't always interact with others as we expect to be treated and they don't always interact with us as we like to be treated.

So, should we throw out our expectations of ourselves and others altogether? Should we expect nothing from each other at all?

I am not among those who would make this argument. I suspect the vast majority of us live with these basic expectations. We expect them in all our relationships—with family, friends, and strangers. We expect them from our bankers, butchers, police, gardeners, bus drivers, cab drivers, and, in our relationships with our physicians. Your physician can provide guidance, clarity, help with your goals, and overall management of your illness so it's important that the time you spend with him or her is high-quality.

In our search for what the ideal patient–physician relationship might look like, let's examine two models: the paternalistic model and the collaborative model.

PATERNALISTIC MODEL: THE OLD SCHOOL

In the old way of thinking among doctors—and often those they served—there was an assumption that the doctor was the one in control, with all of the power, and that the patient was merely subordinate to this all-knowing authority figure. Limited input was solicited from the patient at doctor visits, and patient questions may have been treated as a nuisance. I believe that the following statement sums up this paternalistic attitude: "Do what I say without questioning, and things will be fine." Or, in an offshoot of the classic movie *Tarzan the Ape Man*, "Me doctor, you patient." (Although in reality this phrase was not used in the movie!)

This paternalistic model may still have its place in healthcare, especially in situations involving emergencies or when faced with minor, acute illnesses.

For example:

- If I am severely injured in an automobile accident, I want a trauma surgeon and team who can successfully put me back together again without deferring to me or my family for advice.

- If I need an emergency cardiac bypass, I want a surgeon who can make that happen, quickly and expertly.

- If my heart stops suddenly, I want an Emergency Room physician and team who can quickly restart it.

- If I have strep throat, a sprained ankle, or a bad rash, I would like it treated correctly and quickly by a competent physician. I don't need a lot of consultation; let's just get the job done.

At these moments, most of us would care about little else but recovering. But, when the emergency is over, when the incision is closed, when the defibrillator is shut down—when we are seeing the doctor for continuing care on a chronic illness such as asthma—we want to work with a doctor who encourages us to ask questions and give input. We want to feel comfortable expressing concerns and mentioning solutions for consideration. In short, we want to go way beyond "me doctor, you patient."

Thus, the paternalistic approach works fine for uncomplicated or urgent problems that are brief in duration, but not so much when you are dealing with chronic diseases.* In this book, we are not talking about working in the space of acute life-threatening problems, though we know that asthma can cause acute issues. We are most commonly discussing strategies aimed at helping you beat, or better control, your asthma. We are dealing with chronic illness. I believe that a different model— the collaborative model—is needed. What does this model look like? Let's explore...

THE COLLABORATIVE MODEL

In the collaborative relationship model, equality reigns. I believe that most allergists successfully use the collaborative model.

What do I mean by "equality reigns"? When it comes to dealing with asthma, the ideal relationship is one in which both patient and physician bring their own strengths and expertise to bear on the problem. As an allergist, I bring my knowledge and experience as an asthma expert. As a patient, you bring expertise in yourself, your history, and your observations of

---

* Even in these brief interactions, however, the expectations I listed after the first paragraph above should be met.

your illness. Each of us has an equally important role to play in this relationship.

This is a big shift from the old paternalistic model. This is a shift that all of us will likely welcome!

What might you expect in such a collaborative relationship, beyond the fact that your physician should have a strong foundation of knowledge of asthma? What are the characteristics that you and your physician bring into a relationship that is collaborative in nature? Let's look at physicians first. Collaborative physicians bring the following.

Excellent listening skills. A collaborative physician will really listen to you. I have heard stories from patients who say, "I walked into the doctor's office and he was already writing up a prescription before I'd even spoken," or "She wasn't even interested in what I had to say." What you have to say is extremely valuable, and if your doctor doesn't listen to you, he or she will not be able to help you best manage your asthma, because your valuable input will be missing.

Of course, your doctor has plenty to say, and you are interested in hearing it. But let us not forget that while someone is talking to you, they are not able to listen. Does your doctor give you time to ask questions and give input? Is there any space in your appointments during which the physician just listens?

Physicians learn the importance of taking a good history from a patient very early in their training. This skill first and foremost involves hearing your story. Others might rank it differently, but I put this skill of listening up at the top of the priority list.

Excellent communication skills. As all physicians, I have spent a good portion of my life learning what might be called medicalese or the language of medicine. Although medical jargon serves us physicians well when we are communicating with members of the healthcare team, this jargon has no place when we are communicating with patients or their families.

To be most helpful, an interaction with a physician should be jargon-free and explained in clear and simple terms. I find myself slipping along these lines on occasion and I will either catch myself in the error or my patient may get a perplexed look and ask me to repeat what I have said in plain English, and I shift back into the correct communication mode immediately!

Open and non-judgmental attitude. The collaborative physician creates an open and safe environment where anything can be shared. He or she should be open to hearing what patients see, feel, hear, and do. In the current information and technology age, patients are able to gather reams of information about any topic. If you as the patient see, hear, or read something about asthma, you should be able to bring this information to your physician and discuss it without fear. As an example, if a friend suggests you get a Chihuahua as a pet because it will help your asthma, asking your physician his or her thoughts about this without fear is a reasonable expectation. (You never know till you ask!) You have a right to feel comfortable checking in on this or any other point with your doctor. Free and open exchange of information without fear of judgment should guide the patient–physician relationship.

Honesty. An honest physician will tell you what you need to hear, good or bad. At times, you may hear things that you don't want to hear or that might be upsetting. Your physician needs to have the courage to tell you the truth. If you are to truly collaborate, both parties need to know where they stand at any given time. This is not possible if your physician only tells you what you want to hear.

Hope. Of course, truth doesn't have to be delivered unkindly; it should be framed within a context of hope. Hope has been defined as "the feeling that what is wanted can be had or that events will turn out for the best."[1] In any good patient–physician relationship, the physician will keep hope alive. The belief that better control is possible for the majority of asthmatics is the core belief of this book and may serve as a powerful source of motivation in your own treatment. Medical science marches on. Advances are steadily made. Diseases that seemed hopeless a few years ago can now be successfully treated or prevented. (Think of HIV, polio, or tuberculosis for example.)

Although we need to be honest as physicians, it makes no sense for us to destroy hope. Doing this can be a self-fulfilling prophecy. Have we all not heard of medical cases where all hope was lost, and then the patient went on to recover completely?

Empathy. When it comes to chronic illnesses, a physician functions best when he or she has an appreciation for what patients are experiencing. An empathetic doctor understands that you have fears, that you may have financial and relationship challenges, that you have a life that continues on—in spite of your asthma—with standard everyday stresses and strains. The empathetic doctor understands that we all make mistakes, that we all are fallible, and that things don't always go as the book says they should. For example, you might not recognize the signs and symptoms that your asthma is acting up; or you might forget your medicine or miss appointments. An empathetic doctor will understand that you are a human being and that these things happen. In my mind, understanding and forgiveness go hand in hand with being empathetic. This empathy will keep the patient–physician relationship from being sidetracked and will keep it focused on the common goal of improving asthma control for you.

Now that we know what a collaborative physician looks like, let's look at what collaborative patients bring to the table.

Honesty. Sometimes patients will tell me what they think I want to hear, true or not. In reality, what I need to hear is the plain truth. When we are engaged in making decisions about your care, only complete honesty is helpful.

Recently, for example, I was seeing an adolescent young man for asthma reevaluation. He was continuing to have problems with his asthma, despite the addition of an inhaled steroid inhaler several weeks before. He reported that he was taking his new medication as directed. I was a little suspicious of this, and asked some pointed questions. Feeling some pressure, he explained that he was only using this medication once a day, not twice daily as we had discussed. The truth was critically important here. Why? Because his asthma was still not controlled, I was considering adding a second medication to his daily regimen. This medication came with its own risks to which he would have needlessly been exposed. The cost of care would have been higher and his daily medication routine would have become even more complicated.

This patient's honesty allowed us to address his adherence to the first medication and prevent the needless addition of another medication to the mix. Problem solved. He went on to do much better simply by using the first medicine as required for full and successful effect. When the examination room door closes and it's just patient, physician, and nursing staff, honesty is the best approach.

Self-awareness. You are the expert in your own body. Self-awareness makes this true. If you are aware of the things that are happening to you and the signals your body is conveying, you can then relay this information to your physician. Without this awareness, beating asthma becomes much more difficult.

Some patients can detect very early that their asthma is about to act up when the skin on the front of their neck begins to get itchy. Others know that if there is a certain sound to their cough that an asthma attack is on its way. If you are able to identify and tune in to your particular asthma warning signs, you can give yourself an inside path to staying ahead of problems.

Ownership. I am always concerned when I work with a patient and I am taking his or her asthma more seriously than the patient is. Remembering that this is your disease and that you are ultimately responsible for it is extremely important. No one should take it more seriously than you do. No one should care about how it affects your life more than you.

When you take ownership of your disease, you are also committing to maintaining your effort—persisting. We will talk more about the importance of persistent effort in the next chapter.)

With an attitude of ownership, you are able to enter into a true collaborative relationship with your physician.

Trust. It is true that your sense of trust in the physician will develop (and be earned) over time. Yet, from the start you need to feel some natural degree of trust with the physician to be successful. Without trust, you are more apt to ask someone else for treatment advice.

By working with a physician you naturally trust, you will be able to take the physician's sound medical advice when it is provided to you. Instead of questioning and doubting, you will listen, evaluate, and consider. In this collaborative relationship, trust should continue to grow over time, strengthening the patient–physician bond as it does.

So, we've examined the important characteristics that, in my experience as a physician, are important for both parties to bring to and cultivate in their relationship. This is not meant to be an exhaustive list. You may see some things that are important to you that I have not listed here. You can add or take away from this list to make it yours.

The important concept to remember from this chapter is that serious thought must be given to what you want and expect from your relationship with your doctor. What would you like this relationship to look like so it works for you and your situation? I am confident in your ability to do your part in making this relationship something that serves you well in your quest to beat asthma.

It would be way too bold of me to suggest that I have all the answers. I don't. The framework in this chapter is meant to serve as a guide. I am reminded of the difficulty of accurately defining the collaborative relationship. It reminds me of a statement made by U.S. Supreme Court Justice Potter in 1964 when hearing a case on obscenity. He said: "I shall not today attempt further to define the kinds of material I understand to be embraced...[b]ut I know it when I see it."[2]

So it is with the powerful collaborative relationship between patient and physician. It can be described at length, but, most importantly, you will recognize it when you see it. Of this, I am certain. And, if you do not find it at first, keep looking. Not all physicians are interested in this type of relationship. You have to be ready and willing to fire the doctor who is not collaborative and find one who is. Oftentimes, relatives or friends are a great source of information to help you in your search. Hang in there until you find the right physician for you!

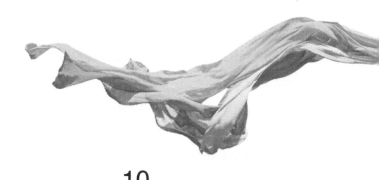

10

Positive Mindset

D o you recall that old expression, "When life gives you lemons, make lemonade"? What does this saying mean to you?

I see it as a recommended reaction to an unfavorable life event. That is, when life gives you lemons (bad circumstances, bad events, difficulties, trials, or whatever you wish to call them), the recommended response is to make lemonade (to turn the bad situation into something positive or to make the best of it). I believe that this saying summarizes well the concept of having a positive mindset—and I believe that having a positive mindset is incredibly important when managing your asthma.

It is important to note here that there is a dearth of research available on the role of positive mindset and improving asthma control. I am largely relating to you what I have observed anecdotally, that is, from my own clinical experience with patients over the past thirty years. Academicians and my fellow physicians may frown upon this suggestion because I have not scientifically studied it, and their skepticism is understandable. But, I am simply telling you what I know to be true from my own observations as food for thought for you.

Hopefully, the scientific proof will come in time based upon the groundbreaking work of people like academic psychologist and author, Dr. Martin Seligman from the University of Pennsylvania. Dr. Seligman could arguably be called the father of positive psychology. Certainly, he is currently its most well-known and respected leader.

What is positive psychology? Just over ten years ago, Dr. Seligman turned away from the pathology and disease-based model of psychology and began to concentrate on human strengths and their role in psychological health and human happiness. This early work has blossomed into a network of psychologists and other relevant professionals and individuals who are looking at understanding the role that human strengths, traits, and characteristics may play in improving education, healthcare, military training, other areas, and society as a whole. If you are interested in learning more about positive psychology, I refer you to Dr. Seligman's books, especially *Authentic Happiness* and *Flourish*, both of which provide a wealth of information on the subject.

What positive traits have I observed in many people who have successfully beaten asthma? In my experience, the positive mindset that arms individuals to do this appears to be composed of three key characteristics: optimism, ownership, and grit. Let's examine each one in more detail.

OPTIMISM

Optimism can be defined as "an inclination to... anticipate the best possible outcome," whereas *pessimism* has been described as "an inclination to emphasize adverse aspects, conditions, and possibilities or to expect the worst possible outcome."[1]

In brief, optimists expect the best; pessimists, the worst. In my observations, asthmatics who are optimistic seem to be able to get their asthma under better control than those who are not. You might ask, did the optimism really come first, or did improved asthma control instead *produce* a more optimistic outlook? It's a valid question. I honestly don't know the answer.

As I said earlier, we have not attempted to measure the relationship between optimism and positive treatment outcomes in our medical practice. Yet, I have certainly seen, firsthand, people come in with poorly controlled asthma who were fed up with the roller coaster ride, yet who *somehow had a glimmer of hope—an idea that things could be much better.* These people appear to be optimistic, and most times we are able to improve their asthma. Their hope leads them to take positive action to find a better way.

I can still recall the mom of one of my patient's, who believed from the very beginning of our work together that we could make things better for her son's asthma. Although I can't be sure, this attitude of optimism (and her approach of wanting to do whatever it took) seemed to make it easier for her to jump right in to supporting the recommended treatment program. Her expectation of hope seemed to give her the mental and physical energy needed to stay on top of her son's treatment. Before long and with the right treatment measures, her son's asthma radically improved: there were no more Emergency Room visits, and office appointments were needed less often.

In contrast, I sometimes meet patients and parents who are feeling pessimistic or low on hope. In situations like these, it sometimes takes more time for me to help these individuals grow comfortable buying into the recommended treatment plan before we see progress.

For example, the pessimist may try the asthma medication for a week, and then give up, thinking, "It won't help anyway," or "I'm not improving so I might as well stop." But as we know from Chapter 3, it can take time for asthma to improve! Optimism may be the bridge to help a patient stick with treatment in order to get those sought-after results.

How so? Optimism can lead to a positive spiral in which hope leads to the willingness and energy to try something new. Those efforts fuel positive improvement in asthma, and more optimism results. With that, the optimism–improvement cycle begins again.

Although research still needs to be done investigating a possible relationship between optimism and asthma control, we know at least that having optimism has been found to be associated with positive health outcomes, even though we are not certain as to why.[2]

The good news is this. Just as *helplessness* is learned, there are techniques that can be applied to improve an individual's optimism and hope. In *Authentic Happiness*, Dr. Seligman outlines a method for establishing optimism that consists of first recognizing, and then disputing, pessimistic thoughts.[3] He teaches you how to argue with yourself when it comes to disputing your own pessimism. Again I refer you to his books for further information.

What are some reasons for you to have hope and optimism? Asthma is treatable! Therapy exists—it just has to be applied correctly. You do not have to suffer day in and day out from it; you can (and will) get it under control. Just think of the seven principles you are learning in this book. By studying them, you are acquiring the tools you need to take better control of your asthma and, as a result, to improve your quality of life. There truly is light at the end of the tunnel!

Second, scientific progress marches on. Right now, there are hundreds, if not thousands, of medical researchers studying asthma. Also, we are steadily gaining a full understanding of the human genome and genetics. Together, these factors will increase our characterization of asthma and will undoubtedly lead to improved therapies, with fewer side effects, and better outcomes. They will, in turn, lead to an improvement in your quality of life. That is something to feel optimistic about.

OWNERSHIP

People who own things tend to treat them differently than people who don't. As an example, have you ever loaned someone a tool or household object and been unhappy with the way they treated it? When you own something, you realize that you are responsible for it. Any good thing or bad thing that happens to your stuff is directly related to how you treat it. Take care of something with great attention and there is a certain pride of ownership that one feels, not to mention positive results. If you don't own something you may feel less responsible for it.

And so it is with asthma. Your asthma belongs to *you*. *You are responsible for it.* The people I see who are capable of taking ownership of their asthma tend to do better than those who don't. They do better than people who view themselves as victims—who never realize that *they own their asthma*.

This may sound harsh, but this is a crucial step in having a positive mindset.

As a matter of fact, until you really take ownership of your asthma, none of the other things in this book really matter. When you take ownership, you pay attention to the little things: things like the way to avoid asthma triggers, the names and doses of the medications you take, what actions you will take when you become sick, and the importance of having a long-term relationship with the same physician. It is close attention to these details outlined in the seven principles that makes a difference between having asthma that is poorly controlled and beating asthma.

GRIT

Self-discipline is necessary to pay attention to all the things you need to manage when you have asthma. The trait of extreme or maximum self-discipline is known as *grit*. In his book *Flourish*, Seligman describes "grittiness" as "the combination of very high persistence and high passion for an objective."[3]

Grit can be measured and has been shown to

- correctly predict which new candidates to West Point will successfully complete the difficult summer training prior to beginning their first year of study and which ones will drop out

- correctly predict making it to the final round of the Scripps National Spelling Bee (participants with higher levels of grit spend more time practicing)
- correctly predict which University of Pennsylvania psychology majors will get higher grades.

In my experience in caring for asthma patients, those with higher grittiness appear to be more successful in achieving and maintaining better control of their asthma. It appears to me as if those who are passionate about the goal or objective of gaining better control over their asthma—and who are persistent in their efforts—are better equipped than those without these traits.

As an example, I recall one mom and dad this past year who had been in and out of Emergency Rooms with their son, who had uncontrolled asthma. These parents were passionate about getting help so that their son would be well. At our first visit, we stepped up his asthma therapy to include a daily controller medication. At follow-up visits with me three and six months later, the need for emergency visits had completely stopped. The parents were highly compliant with his medications. They did not stop when things got better. They were persistent in their efforts, and life changed for the better.

Another example is a longer-term adult patient of mine, who has had a chronic cough due to multiple causes, one of which is asthma. We had tried numerous medications without significant improvement in her condition, and she was becoming more pessimistic of the value of any new medicine I suggested. Who could blame her? At a follow-up visit this past year, we noted that she had been well for three months. When I asked why she thought this had occurred, her reply was, "I suppose it's because I have been really careful to take my [asthma] medications every day as you suggested." She had, for some reason, become more optimistic about the chance her meds would help, and she was sticking to her treatment plan better than I had seen in the past. Boom! Optimism and persistent efforts made a big difference for her!

Once again, these are my own observations. They seem to intuitively make sense but need to be proven (or disproven) through good clinical research. Nonetheless, making better asthma control a goal that you are passionate about—something that you want to achieve above all else—combined with a healthy dose of self-discipline, will better equip you to persist in your efforts at beating asthma. Staying engaged is important because when you have persistent asthma, it requires persistent effort on your part. As an example, I want to bring forward the story of Andrew and his mom from Chapter 2.

> Andrew's mom thinks about his asthma regularly and never puts it out of her mind completely. Andrew's mom also understands that it's she and Andrew who are responsible for dealing with problems as or before they arise (they "own" the asthma) and that there are things she can do to make sure the asthma doesn't get out of control. She has an optimistic

and positive outlook, and Andrew has adopted the same attitude. As a result, she and Andrew are not victims; they are empowered. They have a positive mindset—an outlook that says, "We can deal with everything as it arises"—that leads them to stay engaged and in control.

You can achieve this positive mindset also! Own your asthma, remain optimistic, and never give up in your efforts. This positive mindset, used in conjunction with all the other principles we have looked at in this book, will lead you to your goal of improving control of your asthma. You will then be truly *beating asthma!*

Conclusion: How the Seven Principles Work

Well, we have come a long way in exploring the Seven Simple Principles.

To be fully effective, the principles require action on your part. Similar to a good relationship between a patient and physician, the powerful relationship between a book and its reader is a *collaborative* one. The book provides the expert information on asthma but knows nothing about you. *You* are the expert on you. Only you know where you stand on the spectrum of asthma control. Only you know which of these steps you are already using and which you aren't.

Make an honest assessment of where you are; then, in conjunction with your physician, begin to make progress in better controlling your asthma. As a result, you will improve the quality of your life.

In this chapter, we look at the case of someone who was able to greatly improve the control of his asthma over time and we will analyze what role the seven principles played in his success. Remember Larry? Let's use his example to review how you might use the seven principles in your own life.

THE SEVEN PRINCIPLES, IN ACTION

Larry was about thirty-three years old when we first met.[*] Much like his father, Larry developed asthma and allergies at a young age. He seemed to outgrow his asthma during puberty. Yet, he again began to have problems with asthma in his mid-twenties. As a result, he had been on a roller coaster ride of uncontrolled asthma for about eight years when we first met.

Larry was caught up in a wicked spiral of several Emergency Room visits each year and had several two- to three-day hospitalizations for asthma attacks as well. I felt bad for him.

Larry was seeking care specifically from an asthma physician. Up until that time, he had rarely seen the same physician twice, which meant that his care was fragmented. He was seeing multiple physicians throughout the year, none of whom communicated with each other regarding Larry's condition, progress, or deterioration.

Also problematic, Larry viewed his asthma as being present only when he had coughing and wheezing that he could not control with a bronchodilator. (Of course, we know from Chapter 3 that asthma can be brewing within a person's

---

[*] In reality, "Larry" is a hybrid of a number of real patients that I have cared for over the years.

lungs, ready to worsen at any moment, even when there are no symptoms.) Lastly, Larry had been waking up multiple times each week with cough due to asthma. He had been using, on average, six canisters of bronchodilator medication every year.

During our work together, Larry learned to see asthma as a chronic condition that was always present even when surface symptoms were absent. He learned about the role of (invisible) inflammation in causing his asthma symptoms and, as a result, he saw the benefit of using an inhaled anti-inflammatory medication every day. Using this daily medicine, his nighttime asthma problems quickly ceased. When these disappeared he continued to use this inhaler daily.

Before long, Larry began to see how a different model of care than what he had been using for his asthma was required: same physician, regular check-ups, and prompt attention to early warning signs of an asthma attack.

Once we got his asthma in good shape, we could begin to uncover other related issues. Larry had been having multiple episodes of sinus infections every year. His history and skin testing revealed significant allergies to grass pollens, dust mites, and cats. It was then that Larry recalled that he had been living with his daughter's cat since she moved into an apartment that did not allow pets *over three years ago!* Realizing the importance of avoiding allergens in controlling asthma, Larry found the cat a new home.

Since dust mite allergy was also playing a role in his asthma, Larry began to institute strict dust mite avoidance measures in his home, such as laundering his bed sheets in hot water and using pillow covers (see Chapter 4 for more ideas). After all this was accomplished, Larry's need for his bronchodilator dropped to twice a week, before exercising, to prevent asthma symptoms.

Also of note, Larry's asthma always became worse during the spring and fall months (due to his allergies to grass pollen), and he still required two courses of oral steroids per year to control his asthma during these times. Allergy shots were begun to treat his grass allergy, and the following year he had fewer symptoms during the grass pollen season.

After several months of following his new care plan, Larry was clearly making excellent progress in improving his asthma control. Where previously he would wait several weeks to see a physician for help, he learned a better way. He learned the Rules of Two (see Chapter 1 for details) so that he could quickly assess whether his asthma was controlled or not at a given time, and he knew—due to his action plan—to see a physician for help *soon after* he developed increasing asthma symptoms. He would now seek help in days, not weeks. As a result, he never again required hospitalization for asthma problems. That was quite a difference from when we first met!

In sum, Larry's journey consisted of learning more about the nature of his underlying problem, preventing problems by avoiding triggers, having a collaborative relationship with an asthma specialist, seeking earlier treatment when problems arose, and taking his medications as prescribed. Together, these things all added up to much better asthma control for Larry. Because he was consistently getting a good night's sleep, was spending less money and time on emergency care, and was not suffering with asthma for months on end, the quality of his life dramatically improved!

You may recognize some of your story in the saga of Larry. Larry demonstrates how the understanding and use of the seven principles outlined in this book can help you in *beating asthma*.

I will not kid you: achieving improved asthma control is not easy for everyone, but it is worth the effort. *You* are worth the effort! There remains a relatively small group (though I would argue that any individuals are too many) of people who are leading difficult lives without hope of improving control at the present time due to the severity of their condition. My prayers are with them. As I said earlier, my hope for them lies in continued advances in the understanding and treatment of asthma that are yet to come, and good use of the many options we have today.

For the vast majority of asthma sufferers—among the 70% or so who are currently living with poorly controlled asthma— there exists great hope. My prayer for each of you is that by understanding and applying the principles discussed in this book, in collaboration with a good physician, your quality of life will improve.

Be kind to yourself!

And remember that you are not alone. Feel free to drop by for a visit at www.beatingasthma.com. I look forward to hearing your story!

Appendices

I have provided some additional information and resources in the following pages. Most contain some web site links. As with so many Internet sites, things may change after this book is published. If you find links that are broken or inactive, please let us know by e-mailing editor@beatingasthma.com. Thanks!

Appendices

Appendix A

Additional Resources

Here are some of my favorite links to additional asthma information/resources. This is not an exhaustive list by any means.

Web Address	Resource
www.beatingasthma. com	Companion website for this book. Additional information, community, blog, and more. Come join us and continue your journey to beat asthma.
www.aanma.org	Website for Allergy & Asthma Network / Mothers of Asthmatics. Full of educational resources, advocacy, newsletters, and more.
www.acaai.org	Website for American College of Allergy, Asthma & Immunology

Table continues...

Web Address	Resource
www.aaaai.org	Website for the American Academy of Allergy, Asthma & Immunology
www.aafa.org	Website for Asthma & Allergy Foundation of America. A great resource for asthma as well as allergic diseases.
www.worldallergy.org	Website for the World Allergy Organization.
www.cdc.gov	Website for Centers for Disease Control. Information on asthma, air pollution, and many illnesses.
www.nhlbi.nih.gov/	Web site for National Heart, Lung and Blood Institute, part of the National Institutes of Health. The "Asthma Guidelines" are published by this entity.
www.lungusa.org	Website for the American Lung Association. Information/ education, research news, and "State of the Air" publications.

Appendix B

Asthma Action Plans: Further Comments and Resources

The most commonly used iteration of the asthma action plan today is the traffic signal system. In this scheme, as your peak flow falls and asthma symptoms rise, you move from controlled to uncontrolled asthma, and you find yourself in the green, yellow, or red zone. Each zone contains its own action steps.

Thinking further about the asthma action plan, I realized that it all boils down to one key question, and that is this:

What actions will you take when you find yourself in the yellow zone?

Am I oversimplifying? I don't believe that I am. Think through this with me, if you will.

Green zone: In the green zone, life is good. Asthma is controlled. Your peak flow is 80% or better of your personal best, and no asthma symptoms are present. The only action necessary is to continue to do what you are doing, taking any daily medications as prescribed, and continue to monitor yourself. As with the green traffic signal, green means go!

Red zone: The red zone, similarly, requires little thinking. You are in distress. Your peak flow is less than 50% of your personal best. You are very short of breath, your bronchodilator medications don't help, and you probably have trouble walking and talking. Your lips or fingernails may be blue or discolored (due to lack of oxygen). As with the red traffic signal, stop!

In addition to taking your bronchodilator medication, you need medical attention. Now. Immediately. And the best way to do this is usually to call 911. Not much thinking needed; this is the time for rapid action. To delay action means to risk death.

Although a sudden asthma attack can move you from the green zone immediately into the red zone, this is not the usual case. Typically you will find yourself in the yellow zone first, and this is why the question I posed earlier is so important.

Yellow zone: Again, what actions will you take in the yellow zone? As with the yellow traffic signal, you must proceed with caution. This part of your asthma action plan must be well thought out beforehand, and executed without delay.

First you must recognize that a problem is beginning. When you enter the yellow zone, quite likely your asthma attack is in its earliest stages, with your peak flow falling between 50% and 80% of your personal best. Cough, wheeze, chest tightness, or shortness of breath is/are present. You may be waking up at night due to asthma, and you can do some, but not all, of your usual activities.

Once you recognize the yellow zone, you take action. (If you are in the presence of one of your asthma triggers, get away from it). Taking two puffs of your bronchodilator (albuterol or levalbuterol) or using your nebulizer is the first action step. If you quickly return to the green zone, great, follow your green zone actions. If you don't return to green, your next actions are very important. You really should plan these ahead of time with your physician. Different options are available.

One approach would be to take your bronchodilator inhaler or nebulizer every twenty minutes for an hour and then reassess. If you return to the green zone, continue green zone actions. If not, notify your physician. She or he may have you start a course of oral corticosteroids to help. (If my patients find themselves in the yellow zone for a day or two at the longest, I like to see them in the office). If at any time you worsen (i.e., go to the red zone), you must then take the red zone actions without delay.

I hope my points about the importance of the steps you take in each zone are of some help. The green and red zone actions are pretty straightforward. The yellow zone in asthma, just like the yellow traffic signal, means "caution," proceed with care.

A number of organizations provide asthma action plan templates for your use, including the Allergy & Asthma Networks/Mothers of Asthmatics, Allergy & Asthma Foundation of America Texas Chapter, Centers for Disease Control, and the National Heart, Lung and Blood Institute. Links to these asthma action plans can be found at www.beatingasthma.com.

Appendix C

Tools to Evaluate
Your Asthma Control

1. The Rules of Two®*

As noted earlier in this book, the Rules of Two is a brief, effective tool to determine whether your asthma is out of control and needs medical attention. Simply answer four questions! (I have added the word bronchodilator in italics to be consistent with my text in the book).

Do You:

- Have asthma symptoms or take your quick-relief inhaler *(bronchodilator)* more than Two times a week?

- Awaken at night with asthma symptoms more than Two times a month?

---

* Used with permission of Baylor Health Care System. Special thanks to Carolyn Hicks for her help, as well as Dr. Mark Millard and Mary Hart of the Martha Foster Lung Care Center at Baylor in Dallas, Texas.

- Refill your quick-relief inhaler *(bronchodilator)* more than Two times a year?
- Measure your peak flow at less than Two times 10 (20%) with asthma symptoms?

If you answered "yes" to any of these questions, it appears as if your asthma is not well controlled, seek expert medical advice.

2. Asthma Control Test

This is a simple, several-question survey, with two types based upon age (one for adults and one for children). Based on your score, you can determine whether your asthma has been well controlled or not over the past four weeks. This tool can be found at: http://www.asthma.com/index.html

Look for "Toolbox," then click and take the test!

Appendix D

When to See an Allergist

I am often asked the question, "When should I see an allergist for help with my asthma?"

There are published recommendations providing guidelines to *physicians* as to when to refer a patient to an allergist. Here I would like to provide you with some things for *you* to consider when you ask yourself that question.

SHOULD I SEE AN ALLERGIST?

- Have you had a life-threatening asthma attack?
- Do you have symptoms of asthma during the day and night?
- Does your asthma interfere with your activities of daily living?
- Have you had to stay in a hospital because of asthma?
- Do you have co-existing conditions such as severe hay fever or sinusitis?
- Do you need help to identify asthma triggers?

- Do you need additional help and instruction on treatment plans and medicines?
- Do you think you have allergic triggers that might be helped by allergy shots?
- Does your asthma require oral corticosteroid therapy or high-dose inhaled corticosteroids?
- Have you had to take oral corticosteroids more than twice in one year?

This may not be a complete list, but these are nonetheless the most important questions you should ask yourself. Answering "yes" to any of them means that you should strongly consider seeing an allergist for help in controlling your asthma!

A few final points:

An asthma specialist is also recommended for children ages 0–4 who have asthma symptoms every day and 3–4 nights or more a month. Seeing a specialist also should be considered for children who have symptoms 3 days or more a week and 1–2 nights a month.

The NIH Guidelines for referral to an asthma specialist are in general accord with recommendations of the American College of Allergy, Asthma and Immunology (ACAAI); the American Academy of Allergy, Asthma and Immunology (AAAAI); and the Joint Council of Allergy, Asthma and Immunology (JCAAI), and are endorsed by the Allergy-

Immunology Subsection of the American Academy of Pediatrics (AAP).

The recommendations of these professional medical societies further state that referral to a specialist is indicated when:

- the diagnosis of asthma is in doubt
- the patient asks for a consultation.[1]

Appendix E

How to Use Asthma Inhalers

All too often, I believe that asthma inhalers are prescribed by physicians without providing you, the patient, proper instructions on how to use them. I have searched the net for good resources to help you understand the correct method(s), and listed them below. Remember, if things are still not clear, review your technique with your physician! This is not a complete list but it is a good starting place!

1. The Cleveland Clinic Website

One of America's premier health care systems has provided excellent instructions, not only on using the typical metered-dose inhalers, but on proper use of other delivery systems as well.

http://my.clevelandclinic.org/devices/inhalers/hic_
how_to_use_a_metered_dose_inhaler.aspx

2. The National Institutes of Health's MedlinePlus Website

As described under the "About" tab on the site, "MedlinePlus is the National Institutes of Health's Web site for patients and their families and friends. Produced by the National Library of Medicine, it brings you information about diseases, conditions, and wellness issues in language you can understand. MedlinePlus offers reliable, up-to-date health information, anytime, anywhere, for free." It also provides an easy to understand guide to using inhalers with an open mouth technique. This is a website with a lot of good content!

http://www.nlm.nih.gov/medlineplus/ency/presentations/100200_8.htm

3. National Jewish Health

Located in Denver, Colorado, National Jewish, along with the University of Colorado Hospital, has been named the #1 Respiratory Hospital in the United States by *U.S. News and World Report*. I like their robust educational site because it also has links to YouTube videos that show how to use inhalers.

http://www.nationaljewish.org/healthinfo/medications/lung-diseases/devices/metered-dose/

Notes

CHAPTER 1

1. Sanders, Nancy (President of Allergy & Asthma Network/ Mothers of Asthmatics) and Scott Weiss, MD (Advisors), "Asthma in America" survey (GlaxoSmithKline, 1998).

2. National Heart, Lung, and Blood Institute, "Asthma Guidelines," http://www.nhlbi.nih.gov/health/prof/lung/ asthma/naci/asthma-info/asthma-guidelines.htm).

CHAPTER 2

1. Foggs, Michael B., MD, and Bradley E. Chipps, MD, "Asthma Management and the Allergist: Better Outcomes at Lower Cost," (American College of Asthma, Allergy, and Immunology [ACAAI], 2009).

2. The "Asthma Guidelines" are a publication from an expert panel convened by the National Heart, Lung and Blood Institute in 1991, 1997, 2002, and most recently in 2007, for the care of patients with asthma.

CHAPTER 4

1. Mission Allergy, Inc., "Pillow and Mattress Encasings," http://www.missionallergy.com/?fuseaction=page. display&page_id=60 (accessed August, 12, 2011).
2. Humane Society of the United States, "U.S. Pet Ownership Statistics," http://www.humanesociety.org/issues/pet_overpopulation/facts/pet_ownership_statistics.html (accessed May 14, 2011).
3. Retrieved from http://www.acaai.org/allergist/liv_man/trigger_avoidance/Pages/default.aspx

CHAPTER 6

1. Szefler, Stanley J., et al. "Management of Asthma Based on Exhaled Nitric Oxide in Addition to Guideline-Based Treatment for Inner-City Adolescents and Young Adults: A Randomised Controlled Trial," *The Lancet* 372, no. 9643, doi:10.1016/S0140-6736(08)61448-8.

CHAPTER 7

1. Nelson, Harold MD, et al. "Safety of Formoterol in Patients With Asthma: Combined Analysis of Data From Double-Blind, Randomized Controlled Trials," *The Journal of Allergy and Clinical Immunology* 125, no. 2 (2010), 390–96.e8.

2. American College of Allergy, Asthma, and Immunology, "Efficacy and Safety of Immunotherapy," http://www.acaai. org/allergist/allergies/Treatment/allergy-immunotherapy-shots/Pages/are-allergy-shots-effective.aspx (accessed June 18, 2011).

3. Joint Task Force on Practice Parameters, American Academy of Allergy, Asthma and Immunology, American College of Allergy, Asthma and Immunology, Joint Council of Allergy, Asthma and Immunology, "Summary Statement #69: Allergen Immunotherapy: A Practice Parameter Second Update," *Journal of Allergy and Clinical Immunology* 120, Suppl. 3 (2007), S25–85.

CHAPTER 9

1. Retrieved from http://dictionary.reference.com/browse/Hope?o=100074.

2. Retrieved from http://library.findlaw.com/2003/May/15/132747. html#edn1.

CHAPTER 10

1. Retrieved from http://dictionary.reference.com/browse/pessimism.

2. Zanni, Guido R. "Optimism and Health," *The Consultant Pharmacist* 23, no. 2 (2008), 112–126.

3. Seligman, Martin. *Authentic Happiness: Using the New Positive Psychology to Realize Your Potential for Lasting Fulfillment* (New York, NY: Free Press, 2003), 93–101.

APPENDIX D

1. Foggs, Michael B., MD, and Bradley E. Chipps (Editors), "Asthma Management and the Allergist: Better Outcomes at Lower Cost" (American College of Allergy, Asthma & Immunology, 2009), p. 5.

Acknowledgements

As I write this, I am filled with gratitude. For too many years, this book was just an idea in my mind. While we might agree that good ideas are wonderful, unless they result in action, they remain just that, only good ideas. As I see it, good ideas or intentions alone never help anyone; they need to be accompanied by some type of action.

I finally moved from *thinking* about writing this book to really *beginning* the process in November 2010. While enrolled as a student in the Executive Coaching program at University of Texas, Dallas (UTD), during one of our practice sessions, a fellow student coached me through the idea of writing *Beating Asthma*. Within a 45-minute session, the stumbling blocks I had thrown up in the past were all but gone. I developed a plan to begin and never looked back. That's how we got here today! I am a true testimony to the power of good coaching, and I want to thank Meg Rentschler (who supervised that group) and my fellow students at UTD for their help and support!

I may have had the inspiration to write this book and then weave the words together, but there have been many other people who played a large part in bringing this book to life.

Hillary Clinton once wrote that, "It takes a village to raise a child." These words ring just as true when that "child" is a book, and especially for me, when that book is *Beating Asthma*. To paraphrase Hillary, it takes a village to produce a book! There are many people to thank. I will do my best to recognize them all, and any omissions that may occur are unintended and the fault of my less than perfect brain. So, mea culpa in advance, for any forgetfulness on my part!

The first person I want to thank is my wife, Anne-Marie Apaliski, RN. Her tireless work helped me get through college and medical school. Since I began work on the book, she has been supportive and caring, making sure I took a break when I needed it, understanding the considerable time that has been spent thinking about, researching, and writing this book.

I have always been a reader, for as long as I can recall. I believe it would be difficult to write if you have not, in some form, been a student of the written word. There are two women to recognize for this gift. The first is my mom, Hannah. Although she never completed high school, part of her daily routine was to read the newspaper. Every day. Her modeling of this behavior greatly influenced me and was the beginning of my love affair with books and reading. She passed away when I was only fifteen years old. Thank you, mom. Secondly, I owe tribute to my first grade teacher, Mrs. Ogin. I fondly recall the reading circles we had in her classroom, and how, with her encouragement and instruction, I was able to develop my reading skills. What positive feelings of mastery this led to! Thank you, Mrs. Ogin.

I have been a physician now for just over thirty years as I write this. This journey began for me as a student at the University of Scranton in 1973. I owe a great debt, which I could never repay, to Fr. Bernard McIhlhenny, S.J., who at that time was the Dean of Admissions. He gave a young man a chance to prove himself and allowed him to succeed. He, as well as all of his fellow Jesuits and lay professors, provided a rich, positive, supportive learning environment for me and many other students. Thank you, Father McIhlhenny!

I owe a debt of gratitude to Dr. Michael Kaliner for his review and for writing the foreword for this book. There are so many other people to yet thank, including, professionally, Dr. T. F. McNair Scott, who was a role model when I was a young student at Hahnemann Medical College, as was Dr. Thomas K. "Tim" Oliver (Chairman of Pediatrics at Children's Hospital of Pittsburgh when I trained there), Dr. J. Carlton Gartner, Dr. Paul Gaffney, Dr. Phil Fireman (my earliest allergy and asthma professor), and my fellow Pediatric Residents from 1981–1984, especially my friend and an outstanding Pediatrician, Dr. Paul Dubner.

Special thanks to Nancy Sander, who, through her honest feedback made this a better work, and Drs. Bob Lanier, William E. Berger, Leonard Bielory, Michael Blaiss and Phil Lieberman for your time, support, friendship, and wisdom!

I have been blessed to be the father of two wonderful human beings, Christopher and Sarah, who have kept me young and thinking, just to try to keep up with them. Thanks, kids!

Luckily, I was able to meet Bob and Suzanne Murray from StyleMatters in Philadelphia in October 2010. You guys have been there every step of the way in birthing this book, and I will always remain grateful. Suzanne, with her outstanding editing skills and nurturing personality, has managed to make my writing look and sound good!

I also need to thank and acknowledge my fellow physicians at the Allergy & Asthma Centres of the Metroplex, Drs. C. David Meadows (for his support and mentorship over the past 18+ years), Harry Earl, Neil Singhania, Ted Sugihara, and Drew Beaty. Every physician should be able to have the experience of working with such fine physicians as you. The entire staff at Allergy & Asthma Centres works tirelessly to help our many patients deal with asthma. To Shirley Grooms, practice manager, and Kit Owings, R.N., chief nurse, I owe my undying gratitude. You gave the "new guy" a chance. Thanks. It has been an interesting ride. To Jan Baker, Tara Shook, Teresa Leonard, Brandi Murley, Carol Lewis, Brenda Fowler, Lori Cortinas, Elizabeth Grainger, Barbara Kelley, LeeElla Anderson, Pola Simon, Becky French, Sylvia van Leemput, Debra Eaton, Jaime Jones, Julie Clay, and Ashley Bermingham,

I extend my deepest thanks. It is an honor to work with such a great team.

Thanks also to good friends Jerry, Rick Colleoni, Carolyn Costello, PhD, Mike Neuland, MD, David Young, MD, Scott Holliday, MD, John F. McCracken, PhD, Dr. and Mrs. Vince Grattolino, and my dearest cousins David and Joan Winters

Perhaps most importantly, I want to thank the many patients and families I have been blessed to work with over the past thirty years. A doctor learns many things from books but can only become a good physician by taking care of people and by caring for people. I believe that, over the years, I have learned more from you than you have learned from me. Watching so many of you win the battle, moving from uncontrolled to controlled asthma, has been my inspiration in writing this book. I know that what you have done, others can do. May your successes inspire them all. Thank you everyone!

Stephen J. Apaliski, MD
Colleyville, Texas
September 2011

About the Author

D r. Apaliski has been a practicing physician for over 30 years. He first trained as a pediatrician at the Children's Hospital of Pittsburgh and later as an allergist at Wilford Hall United States Air Force Medical Center in San Antonio, Texas. In 1990, he served as a flight surgeon in the first Gulf War.

Dr. Apaliski is Board Certified in Pediatrics as well as Allergy & Immunology. In addition, he is a Fellow of the American College of Allergy and Immunology and a Board Member of the Allergy and Asthma Foundation of America—North Texas chapter. He is also certified by the Association of Clinical Research Professionals as a Certified Physician Investigator.

In addition to seeing patients in his medical practice at the Allergy & Asthma Centers of the Metroplex and conducting Clinical Trials as the Medical Director of Discovery Trials-Arlington, Dr. Apaliski is on the medical staff at THR Arlington Memorial Hospital in Arlington, Texas.

Dr. Apaliski is also a speaker for various Pharmaceutical Companies, helping to educate physicians and other health care providers about the diagnosis and treatment of asthma and allergic diseases.

Dr. Apaliski has two children and resides in Colleyville, TX, with his wife.

9 780984 876907